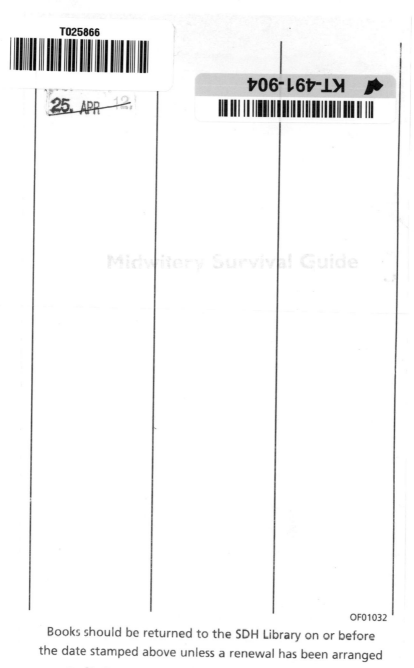

Other Quay Books titles in midwifery include:

Birth Stories for the Soul
Birthing Positions
Care for Obese Pregnant Women
Challenges for Midwives Vol 1
Demystifying Qualitative Research in Pregnancy
Essential Guide for Student Midwives
HIV and Midwifery Practice
Maternal Infant Nutrition and Nurture
Miscarriage
Perineal Care
Psychology for Midwives
Sociology for Midwives
Statutory Supervision for Midwives

Series editor
Dr John Fowler

Note

Healthcare practice and knowledge are constantly changing and developing as new research and treatments, changes in procedures, drugs and equipment become available.

The author and publishers have, as far as is possible, taken care to confirm that the information complies with the latest standards of practice and legislation.

Midwifery
Survival Guide

by

Jacqui Williams

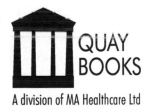

QUAY
BOOKS

A division of MA Healthcare Ltd

Quay Books Division, MA Healthcare Ltd, St Jude's Church, Dulwich Road, London
SE24 0PB

British Library Cataloguing-in-Publication Data.
A catalogue record is available for this book.

ISBN-10: 1-85642-412-X
ISBN-13: 978-1-85642-412-7

Cover design by Louise Cowburn, Fonthill Creative
Publishing Manager: Andy Escott

Printed by CLE, Huntingdon, Cambridgeshire

Contents

Preface

What will it be like to be a newly-qualified midwife? Reaching this milestone achievement really brought out mixed feelings in me. I was so pleased and proud to have got through the 3 years of training (plus an interruption) and to have finally qualified. Then the NMC sent me my PIN and that's when it really sank in.

The PIN meant that it wasn't a dream, or I wasn't being strung along — it had actually happened. I also had a job to go to at my training Trust. This was the point at which I started thinking about the responsibility that comes with the job, and it's fair to say that a healthy amount of fear started to creep in. I hoped I would be a good midwife — that I would do no harm, advocate for the women I cared for and generally keep up with everything, my family included (without their support I wouldn't have qualified in the first place). I finally accepted that I was a qualified midwife when the midwives I was working with saw me and said, 'Oh, look at you in your uniform! Well done!'

On starting my job, there was a month's induction period, during which all of us who were starting jobs within the Trust attended compulsory training days. These covered obstetric emergencies, where to get our passwords, how to fill in extra duty forms (very important), and there was further training on epidurals, suturing and administering drugs — we all passed a test to enable us to do drug rounds on the ward. It was a very full-on month, but training took place during office hours and most of my cohort was kept together for teaching. We all went to various clinical areas for a couple of days' induction here and there.

At the end of the month, each of us was allocated our rotation — that is, the clinical area we would work in for the first few months before moving around the hospital to other areas. Mine happened to be the delivery suite. I am so glad I went there first as until this point, I had never been unsupervised or on my own in a room at a birth — for every other minute around that point yes, but not for the birth itself. I was daunted to say the least, but as you may hear people say, it is a bit like gaining confidence after passing your driving test. Everybody is uncertain of something, and needs experience of it in the driving seat.

My Trust provided a preceptorship period of about 3 months. Due to the busy nature of midwifery units, your allocated preceptor may not be working the same shifts as you or even working in your area, so much of making contact and getting together will be self-directed. At the very least, there is an experienced midwife who you can go to and ask questions.

The first year following qualification has a steep learning curve. You will gain experience, learn new skills and clinical procedures and learn to care for women. Prep creeps in too, as you continue to write reflections on experiences you have been in and learnt from or wish to learn from. You must remember to request days off and annual leave far enough in advance that it is possible, not forgetting that if something crops up, swapping shifts with colleagues means that one of you can't work.

I found my cohort who stayed on at the unit to be brilliant support — friends I was able to discuss things with that no one else would have understood. Wherever you work, the other midwives will soon become good friends as you settle in. Although people don't often say it out loud, everybody has crises of confidence. It's not just you. If you need help, ask for it. If you need support, ask for it — it's there. Also, a book like this will be really helpful during the third year of the midwifery programme and in the first year of practice — quick and easy to dip into if you have a query.

The 'newly-qualified' part of being a midwife seems to stop when the cohort beneath you in training qualify, or when you get your band 6 — whichever happens soonest. The thing to remember is that you can do it. You have passed a lot of exams to get to this point. No one is expecting you to be world class on day one. All midwives were newly-qualified at some point and most can remember being so. Being a midwife is one the most rewarding professions in existence, go for it!

Andrea Simpson
Registered Midwife
Student Midwife 2006–2009
De Montfort University
Leicester, 2011

Contributors

Claire Agnew RN(Adult), DipHE Nursing, PGCE, ENB124, ENB 998, Senior Nurse Clinical Practice Development, University Hospitals of Leicester NHS Trust, Leicester.

Rowena Doughty MSc, PGDE, BA (Hons), ADM, RN, RM. Senior Lecturer in Midwifery and Supervisor of Midwives, De Montfort University, Leicester.

Deborah Dowsett MA BA(Hons) DPSN RGN, Senior Lecturer - Nursing, School of Nursing and Midwifery, De Montfort University, Leicester.

John Fowler PhD MA, BA, DipN, CertED, RGN, RMN, RCNT, RNT, Principal Lecturer - Nursing, School of Nursing and Midwifery, De Montfort University, Leicester.

Bernadette Gregory Masters in Midwifery (MMID) BA (Hons) Health Studies Diploma in Adult Education, PGCEA, RM, ADM, Senior Lecturer in Midwifery, De Montfort University, Leicester.

Karen Mee BSc (Hons) (Open) RGN, RM, Post Graduate Certificate Managing Health and Social Care , Supervisor of Midwives, Practice Learning Lead for the Women's and Children's Division, University Hospitals Leicester.

Jethi Modhvadia Bsc (Midwifery) Diploma in Midwifery, Midwife - mainly working and promoting the low risk midwifery area. University Hospitals of Leicester NHS Trust, Leicester

Sue Nyombi Senior Lecturer in Midwifery De Montfort University, Leicester.

Molly Patterson MSc, BA (Hons) RN, RM, Research and Development Midwife, University Hospitals of Leicester NHS Trust, Leicester.

Kevin Power MA, BA(Hons), Dip(N), CertEd, RSCN, RGN, Associate Head of School, School of Nursing and Midwifery, De Montfort University, Leicester.

Andrea Simpson Diploma in Higher Education, RM, Midwife, De Montfort University, Leicester.

Jacqui Williams MA (Distance Education) PGCEA, BSc (Hons) ADM, RGN, RM Senior Lecturer in Midwifery, De Montfort University, Leicester.

Zaheera Essat BSc, PhD, RM, Midwife, University Hospitals of Leicester NHS Trust and part time Midwifery Lecturer, De Montfort University, Leicester.

Chapter 1

Now I am a qualified midwife

'To be eligible to practice as a midwife a person must hold a midwifery qualification, have current registration as a midwife with the NMC, and meet the NMC Standards for updating her midwifery practice. In addition she must have given notice of her intention to practice to the local supervising authority in every area that she intends to practice in.'

'*Midwives Rules and Standards*' (NMC 2004)

- **How do I prepare for an interview for a midwifery post?**
- **How do I adjust to becoming a qualified midwife?**
- **How do I work with others and become part of the team?**
- **How do I manage my time?**
- **How do I get to grips with working unsocial hours?**
- **How do I deal with experienced maternity care assistants?**
- **How can I evaluate midwifery practice?**
- **Working in a research role**

How do I prepare for an interview for a midwifery post?
Claire Agnew/Jacqui Williams

Creating the right impression at interview takes preparation. For some jobs you may be the only applicant. Other jobs may have 10 or 20 applicants for one position. No job will be yours automatically. You need to find ways of getting the edge over other applicants, and this means preparation and presentation.

Getting an interview will depend on your application form, which must be both concise and comprehensive. To give yourself the best chance of being shortlisted ensure your application form addresses the following:

- Do not write in blue ink when your application form asks for black.
- Ensure that your handwriting is legible.
- Fill in every section.
- Make sure that the supporting statement box includes personal qualities.
- What have you done outside of work that could have a positive effect on your midwifery practice?
- You should demonstrate insight into the role that you are applying for. Do not simply say, 'I want to work in this unit to increase my skills in normal midwifery care.'
- Articulate that you are motivated and that you will demonstrate commitment to and fit into the team.

Pointers for applying for posts and interviews

If possible, try to make an informal visit before applying for a post. If the role is a potential promotion within your existing area, arrange to see the senior midwife, practice development midwife or midwifery manager. This will give you an opportunity to find out others' expectations of the role that you are applying for and will aid your preparation; it will also demonstrate your interest and commitment. Work on your *curriculum vitae* and application form to ensure that they reflect your suitability for the post.

If you are unsuccessful, try not to be too disappointed. The more sought after or senior the job, the greater the interest and competition will be. Do your best to learn from the experience, in terms of things that you can improve on in future applications and also in terms of character development. Following most interviews there will be the opportunity to receive feedback; if this is not offered to you, then ask. Try to treat this positively and make sure that you are willing to listen, learn and develop.

See the boxes opposite for some top tips for interviews and for some examples of questions that you may be asked at interview.

Top tips for interviews

• Research the role that you are applying for
• Dress smartly — you are a professional
• Read the job description thoroughly and think through what the role involves
• Think of some possible scenarios that you may be asked about; where possible, answer questions with reference to previous experiences that you have learnt from
• Think of some questions to ask the panel — write these down so that you can refer to them if need be
• Take your professional profile with you and offer it to the panel to look at
• Arrive in good time — this will allow you to collect your thoughts.

Questions you may be asked at interview

• Why do you want this post?
• How do you deal with stress?
• What is important to you as a midwife?
• What do you understand by the term 'midwifery supervision'?
• What do you understand by the term 'clinical governance'?
• What do you understand by [insert the name of any current government initiative or publication]?
• What qualities do you possess that you can bring to this role?
• Who or what has most inspired you?
• Tell me about a recent article that you have read, which has influenced your practice.

How do I adjust to becoming a qualified midwife?

Penny Tremayne/Jacqui Williams

Transition: a reality shock

Cast you mind back a few years — can you remember why you wanted to become a midwife? You may have answered the question as follows:

- I want to make a difference to families' lives.
- I want to work as a professional in every sense of the word.
- I want to contribute to society.

Hopefully nothing has changed. As a student midwife, there is a tendency to wish the time away. However, when you first put on the uniform, there is a mixture of emotions — not only are you now visible as a registered midwife, you actually are one. Even the most confident newly qualified midwife may wish to reverse time and return to the safety of being a student. Fear, excitement and anxiety are all normal. You may recall people harping on about 'lifelong learning' at university, and while you will pursue further education, the learning of 'real-life midwifery' begins once you register. A useful analogy is learning to drive — you must achieve a required level of proficiency to qualify, but it is only through experience that you truly develop, refining your skills and adapting appropriately.

So there are differences — yes, you are now professionally accountable, you have a different uniform and likely greater responsibility in the maternity setting that you work in, but the fundamentals of midwifery care have not changed.

What does a midwifery manager expect of a newly registered midwife?

Their expectations are that you will:

- Deliver a high standard of care.
- Be kind and caring to women, their partners and families and to other members of staff.
- Be honest and trustworthy.
- Communicate effectively.
- Demonstrate initiative and use common sense.
- Prioritise your workload.
- Be a good team worker.

- In time, be expected to supervise staff, work as a team leader and delegate work appropriately.
- Be punctual, neat and tidy.

You will already have demonstrated many of these attributes as a student midwife. However, it is likely that you will still feel nervous. You need to be kind to yourself and understand that it is normal to be apprehensive.

Locasto and Kochanek (1989) explain a 'reality shock' that nurse educators go through, and it may be useful to explore this concept to better understand the experience of the newly qualified midwife.

In the 'honeymoon period' (as a newly registered midwife) there is a sense of novelty. No longer dependent on a means-tested bursary, qualification means that you now have a salary and some decent money at long last. The hard work of the previous three years has resulted in its ultimate goal and there is a sense of achievement. Finally, the work setting welcomes you as a part of a team.

However, shock and rejection can follow. Shock comprises five phases:

- **Moral outrage** — newly registered midwives can find the intensity of shifts too much, being asked to come in on 'days off' to cover for sick colleagues, and having to work extended shifts due to staff shortages. Managers often want midwives to take on different roles — what time is there to do that?
- **Rejection** — despite every intention to be 'the best midwife', limited resources, confrontations and frustrations with other staff can make the newly registered midwife feel as though she is a failure. There may be the perception that others are much better.
- **Fatigue** — adapting to the new role can leave newly registered midwives physically and mentally exhausted. Fatigue can impact on their social lives, compromising relationships and leaving them too tired to pursue hobbies.
- **Perceptual distortion** — newly registered midwives can think that they are not working as effectively as their peers and can develop anger towards the maternity setting that they work within. This can be vented at meetings, where contributions can be hyper-critical, superficial and lacking in objectivity. All in all, perceptions can be far too negative. It is as if newly registered midwives are in 'too deep' and in a state of 'shock'.
- **Resolution** — this is the final stage, and refers to recovery or resolution.

During this difficult time, various strategies can help midwives adapt. For instance, the assistance of role models can be helpful. Although many areas have a preceptorship programme, newly registered midwives can also seek solace away from the work setting, with people who are sometimes better able to help them make sense of their situation. Another strategy is to keep a reflective diary, which can then be used to identify issues and to develop and change practice accordingly. Such strategies can reduce the intensity of these midwives' work and as a sense of objectivity dawns, some can even find an amusing side to it all.

A nursing study by Benner (1984) identified five levels of competency in clinical practice, namely: 'novice', 'advanced beginner', 'competent', 'proficient' and 'expert'. In this seminal piece of writing, Benner considers the complexity of nursing; it is acknowledged that proficient nurses will have often worked with a similar patient population for 3–5 years, and that expert nurses frequently have an intuitive grasp of situations. The same can be applied to midwifery practice. You mustn't forget that it is unfair to compare yourself to midwives who are more experienced than yourself. Realise that registration and starting work is a transition that can involve aspects of reality shock. Try to set up strategies that will support you through this time, so that your transition is less 'shock and rejection' and more 'honeymoon and resolution'.

Your co-workers will expect you to ask questions and be in need of support. A small, alphabetically arranged notebook can act as an *aide memoire* and save you having to ask the same questions repeatedly.

Good luck!

How do I work with others and become part of the team?
Karen Jackson/Jacqui Williams

Becoming part of a team

When you qualify, the prospect of becoming part of a team can be daunting — for one thing, all of your colleagues seem to know each other already. You will be keen to make a good impression.

You need to spend some time understanding how your new team works. Who are the core midwives? Which teams of medical staff will you work inter-professionally with? How does the on-call system work? This knowledge is essential if you are to promptly refer to an appropriate professional when you need a colleague to review the woman you are caring for. If you are working within a new trust, you will also need to familiarise yourself with the documentation used.

It is one of your preceptor's duties to introduce you to colleagues and to members of the multidisciplinary team. Do your best to remember their names. Although some people have a knack for this, it can be tricky at first. Name badges and photo boards on the ward may help to jog your memory. It can also help to get to know a bit about your colleagues. For instance, do they have children? What are their hobbies or interests? This knowledge enables you to take an interest in your colleagues — they will often appreciate being asked about particular events, such as a birthday party or their child's first day at school. Knowledge of your colleagues' lives outside of work can also help you to understand why they may, on occasion, not be their usual selves.

You will need to get to know the particular roles and responsibilities of different members of the team. Is there a consultant midwife? Who does the off duty? Who is responsible for students? Who has expertise at screening, or at managing patients with complex needs, such as those with diabetes or who are experiencing bereavement?

You will also need to be aware of any cliques within the team and do your best to avoid being drawn into them. You must tread the fine line between trying to get on with everybody and alienating your colleagues. Keep an open mind to begin with and choose your loyalties carefully. Inevitably, you will find that there are some people that you get on with less well than others. Accept this and focus on being polite, courteous and professional at all times while on duty.

One of the most useful things that you can do is to get to know your ward clerk, if you have one. They are often mines of useful information, with networks of contacts in many areas — they can potentially save you having to make numerous, frustrating phone calls to get things done.

Time management and prioritisation are difficult skills to learn and like so much else in midwifery, will be invisible when done well. A useful starting point for ward-based staff is a sheet of paper highlighting your allocated women, which states what needs doing and when. Are there observations to be made, infusions to be read or observed, or medicines to be given? This sheet gives an hour-by-hour breakdown of your workload in terms of tasks.

You must think about how to organise yourself. Do you really have to go to the same woman three times in the space of 30 minutes, attending to different elements of care? This will be tiring for her and for you, and will add to the distance walked during a shift. When starting in a new area, you should make sure that you can access all the equipment that you will need. Use your first few days to find out where things are kept and how they are ordered.

To make your contact more effective, think about how you can cluster care. You must be mindful of colleagues' workloads when planning your own. For example, it would be unreasonable to present your colleague with a drug chart five minutes before intravenous antibiotics are due, and expect them to drop everything and administer the drugs for you. Such tasks must be discussed at the beginning of the shift, so that your colleagues can manage their own workloads and be aware of the tasks that they have to schedule in.

If and when you are up to date with your work, you should think about how to use your time. Try to avoid sitting at the desk making casual conversation with other staff — while this can be relaxing and useful for short periods of time, there are some useful things that you can be doing. You might offer to help colleagues, or ensure that areas are tidy and that supplies are well-stocked — think how frustrating it is when somebody else has used the last of something and not replaced it. The label 'lazy' is easy to get and extremely difficult to get rid of, so it is best avoided in the first place!

Midwives working in a community setting should be especially mindful of safety, and should ensure that they keep a diary for planning visits, putting scheduled clinics into the diary first and then planning other appointments around them.

Working with others

What do 'leadership' and 'being in charge' mean to you? These are not necessarily the same thing. Think about the people you worked with as a student midwife — what were the leadership skills that you admired in them? Here are some of the things that are considered to be important:

- Fairness in workload allocation (this includes balancing allocations of women in normal labour and those with complex needs).
- A willingness to help others without being asked.
- Noticing when your colleagues are struggling and supporting them, without taking over.
- Taking the lead when the situation demands it, such as in an emergency.

These are key points to consider in terms of your professional development, as through experience and continuing education you will prepare to, ultimately, take a more senior role within the team.

How do I manage my time?

Claire Agnew/Jacqui Williams

As midwives, we spend so much of our professional lives looking after others that it is easy to forget to look after ourselves. It is important to maintain a social life as well as a career. We hope that the following will help you through the working day and point you in the right direction to achieve a happy and healthy career! Ask yourself these questions:

- How many times have I not taken my break to get things done?
- How often do I get off work on time?
- How often do I get home and then phone work to pass on something that I have forgotten?
- How long do I spend looking for things that I have lost or mislaid?

If your answer is 'sometimes' or 'frequently', then you need to develop some time management strategies to help you through the day and to feel that you have achieved your goals by the end of it. Two important aspects of time management are:

- Being more **efficient** (doing things *right*).
- Being more **effective** (doing the *right things*).

The elements of time management include prioritisation, putting things off and delegation. These are detailed below.

Prioritisation

- Make a list of everything that you have to do and keep this with you all day.
- Divide your work into three categories, ranked according to priority:
  1 = urgent and important
  2 = important but less urgent
  3 = routine and low priority.
- As soon as you have completed a task, cross it off your list — nothing is more satisfying than seeing a list of tasks getting shorter.
- Be prepared to re-prioritise – a midwife's work is never static.
- Communicate with your team regularly throughout each shift, so that you all know what is going on.
- Seek help and support from colleagues as soon as you feel that you are getting bogged down with work; never be afraid to ask.
- Only keep one list — any more than this will be confusing.

Putting things off

We put things off because:

- The task is overwhelming and we are frightened of failure.
- We have little or no information to start the task, are indecisive or are unsure of priorities.
- We cannot find things, or are too busy doing unimportant things.
- We may be stressed, ill or suffering from chronic fatigue.

Ways to move forward:

- Tackle the worst or the easiest task first.
- Break tasks up into smaller, manageable chunks.
- Do the parts that you feel you can do first.
- Consider seeking advice to help you complete more challenging tasks.

Delegation

Delegation is an important aspect of time management for a qualified midwife. Reasons to delegate:

- It frees up time for the jobs that only you can do.
- It can allow others to learn new tasks.
- It can motivate colleagues to become more useful members of the team.
- The job may be done better by someone else.

Why we do not delegate:

- We feel that we can do the job better.
- We do the job faster.
- We enjoy doing the job.
- Force of habit.
- We fear letting go, as someone else may do the task better.

The best ways to delegate:

- Choose the person most suitable for the job.
- Ensure that they are capable of performing the task.

- Explain the job and ask them if they foresee any problems.
- Leave them to get on with it.
- On completion of the task, ask them how they got on and help them to deal with any unresolved issues.

(Hindle 1998; Martin 2000)

How do I get to grips with working unsocial hours?

Claire Agnew/Jacqui Williams

Requesting off duty

We all deserve a life outside of work. How often do we hear it said that the off-duty folder rules our lives? This can easily happen when getting to grips with a new job. The average person has many things to juggle throughout their day — work, partners, friends, family and further study — yet looking after your own health and wellbeing remains important.

Be aware that you can make requests for off duty but remember:

- Be fair — your team members would like to have a life as well.
- Plan ahead — there is no point expecting to get the days off you want if you do not go to book them until the week before.
- Most off duty is planned 6–8 weeks ahead.
- Do not go for 4 months without a holiday, or you will be too burnt out to enjoy it.
- Space your annual leave evenly throughout the year.
- Follow any local guidelines for leave requests or self-rostering. You should be able to answer questions such as:
  - How many staff can be off at any one time?
  - Do you need to book the weekend off before annual leave?

Special duty payments

We all know that midwifery is a 24 hours, 7 days a week profession; to work nights, weekends and bank holidays is all part of the job. However, most midwives get some financial reward for working these 'unsocial hours', which can be claimed for by filling in the appropriate forms at your place of work. It is your responsibility to complete any paperwork related to special duty payments, and to ensure that applicable shifts are signed for. You may be asked to sign forms for other members of staff — if you do, it is your responsibility to be certain that they have worked the hours written on the form.

Maintaining a social life while doing shift work

Work should stay at work and home should stay at home, but how easy is this to achieve? The important thing to remember is that it is all about maintaining a balance. Does working a run of 12-hour shifts, doing three nights, having two days off and then starting back again on an early shift sound like a challenge?

It can be difficult to get used to, and it is important that you are fit to function while on duty. You are an accountable practitioner and you must be able to function with off-duty. However, if you find that you are getting regular nine to 10 day stretches or a quick turnaround from days to nights and then back to days, you need to discuss this with your preceptor, mentor, ward sister or line manager.

Becoming tired and stressed through shift work could affect your care, and it is important to recognise this. You must do something positive and seek out support mechanisms.

How do I deal with experienced maternity care assistants?

Karen Jackson/Jacqui Williams

'Qualified maternity support workers/maternity care assistants should be employed within a nationally agreed framework, which defines their role, responsibilities and arrangements for delegation, supervision and makes it clear that their role is to support and not replace the midwife.'

Midwifery 2020 Programme (2010)

You may feel inadequate or threatened if you are responsible for supervising very experienced staff, such as maternity care assistants. Maternity care assistants often have considerable experience and are very familiar with routines. Make sure that you treat everybody with equal respect. If you gain people's respect, you will find that they will work with you and for you. Work hard and enthusiastically and staff will follow your lead.

It may seem obvious, but how you ask people to do things makes a difference — you must do your best to avoid seeming lazy or bossy. A comment about newly qualified midwives often heard from maternity care assistants is that they would be happy to help, if only they were asked in a pleasant manner.

Do not be frightened or embarrassed to ask your colleagues for their opinions and advice. For instance, maternity care assistants spend a lot of time with the women, so make sure to ask them how they think the women are coping— their feedback should be valued. Make sure that you understand how they fit into the team. What is their role?

While you should not be afraid to ask others within the team to help you out, you must recognise when you cannot delegate. The knowledge and experience of maternity care assistants varies considerably — you should not assume that a person is competent to undertake a particular duty, simply because they have worked in that area for two years.

You may feel uncomfortable asking an experienced maternity care assistant if they know how to do something, especially if they are quite a bit older than you are. However, you are the accountable practitioner and it is your responsibility to ensure that the person you ask to perform a task has the necessary skills and knowledge to undertake it safely. In turn, they are responsible for recognising their limitations and for not taking on duties that they are not competent to perform. You need to be aware of what individuals can and cannot do, and of your trust's policy in assessing competence.

How can I evaluate midwifery practice?
John Fowler/Mollie Patterson/Jacqui Williams

'The definition of quality should be further enhanced to take account of all six dimensions of quality: person-centredness, safety, effectiveness, equity, and timeliness together with women's experience and satisfaction with care. Equity should included in a measure of quality to ensure that safety, effectiveness and the experience of women do not vary as a result of factors such as age, ethnicity, area of residence or socioeconomic status.'

Midwifery 2020 Programme (2010)

If we are going to evaluate practice developments, we must ask what it is exactly that we are going to evaluate? Is it our views as midwifery practitioners, the women's views, the managers' views, or maternity outcomes? One of the first rules of evaluation is to be very clear about what it is that you want to evaluate. You must acknowledge that it is not possible to evaluate everything, and that when evaluating just one or two areas (probably from one perspective) there can be other effects that you may or may not recognise. At best, your findings will be a partial evaluation — you must avoid the danger of making claims that cannot be substantiated by your evaluation procedure.

To give an example, when interpreting the findings of the HOOP trial (McCandlish *et al* 1998) — an evaluation of traditional techniques for protecting the perineum during the second stage of labour — it was widely suggested that the 'hands on' approach, which was custom and practice for many midwives, was inconsequential in preventing perineal trauma. This had a significant impact on clinical practice, with many midwives adopting the 'hands poised' technique instead. It was actually concluded that there was no difference in pain at 10 days, whether the perineum was supported or not. However, the study failed to consider differences in perineal trauma between the two groups, as the incidence of 3rd and 4th degree tears was small and it was not sufficiently powered to detect any.

The simplest evaluations are where a single factor has a single effect. For example, you might study acupuncture for the treatment of nausea and vomiting in early pregnancy, with one group receiving acupuncture (intervention group) and the other receiving no acupuncture (control group). There is considerable difficulty when evaluation involves multiple factors.

What is the best method of evaluation?

No one method of evaluation is the best. Each method varies in terms of robustness and depending on the nature of the situation being evaluated, some methods will be more appropriate than others.

Randomised controlled trials (RCTs)

Often referred to as the 'gold standard' of evaluation (Shepperd *et al* 1997), an RCT is a longitudinal study in which participants are randomly selected into two groups — one of which is given the 'treatment' that is being studied and the other, the 'control' group, is given nothing.

Comparisons are then made between the treatment group and the control group. RCTs have varying levels of sophistication, as different designs have different levels of blinding. In simple terms, patients, practitioners and researchers can all be kept unaware of the treatment group that a patient is in, not knowing whether they are receiving the treatment or a placebo. If an RCT is well-designed with the control and treatment groups being as similar as possible, the elimination of all possible bias, the 'treatment' a single or easily identified variable and the outcomes objectively measurable, then the evaluative and predictive power of the RCT cannot be bettered. RCTs are predominantly used with pharmacological treatments, although there are a few examples of their use in surgery and other areas (Shepperd *et al* 1997).

Before and after studies

Before and after studies (Polit and Hungler 1995) are another form of longitudinal study, in which baseline measurements are made prior to a treatment being used and then similar measurements are made following its introduction. The before and after measurements are compared and conclusions are then drawn. A problem with such studies is that during the time period, other variables apart from the treatment can be introduced, 'contaminating' our measurements. Furthermore, over time a number of medical conditions will improve without any external treatment. If we were to conduct a before and after study on patients with back pain, for instance, and the treatment was to put a plaster on each patient's back for four weeks, we would probably find that a significant number of patients would report that their pain had subsided during the study. We might then claim that our treatment — the plaster — had worked. It would not be difficult to exchange this plaster for a more exotic treatment, which might then be marketed and sold.

When mindful of their shortcomings, before and after studies can be useful and will often be used to evaluate a new practice or approach to midwifery. When the results and conclusions are presented within a context of other variables that may have had an influence, these studies can be useful for suggesting general trends and informing views on what effect the 'treatment' has. However, they cannot be used in the same way as a well-designed RCT.

Case studies

Case studies (Bowling 1997) focus on a single person, or example of what is being studied. Following a person over a period of time, they are another example of a longitudinal study. Case studies may incorporate regular measurements or interviews with the subject. They tend to take a more holistic view of the situation, trying to acknowledge and possibly prioritise the various interacting variables that may have affected the person or situation. A case study can involve a single woman or a specific area of midwifery practice, such as the delivery suite. The results and conclusions from case studies can be used to give new and more holistic insights into what is happening in a particular situation. What might have been true in one woman's case might also be relevant to others, or what seemed to work in one delivery suite might also be appropriate in another similar area. However, the emphasis must be on the words 'might be relevant'.

Case studies are particularly useful for giving a holistic picture and also for their ability to identify important variables that may have a significant influence on a situation. Their strength, which is also their weakness, is that they allow human judgement to interact with a complex multi-variable situation, appreciating the holistic nature of the situation as well as identifying possible quirks that may be influencing it.

Surveys

Surveys (Bowling, 1997) take a snap shot of a situation, often using questionnaires or interviews. They will usually begin by identifying a particular group of the population, e.g. pregnant women with diabetes. Using appropriate sampling techniques, a proportion of that group is identified. The sample group is then asked certain questions, usually via a questionnaire or sometimes face-to-face. Alternatively, the survey may involve some form of test, observation or investigation, e.g. antenatal screening. Provided the sample group of women has been randomly selected from the pregnant population, then the results of the survey can be generalised back to the population. Surveys vary considerably in quality, which depends on the degree of randomisation of the sample, the questionnaire's design, response rate, and analysis of the results. They are particularly useful in gaining a general view of a particular group of the population, and are often used to gain woman and midwife satisfaction views.

Working in a research role

Mollie Patterson

First time as a research midwife

The best way to gain your first experience in research is to work on a research study, with a research team made up of academics and clinicians. Research midwives are mainly involved in the collection of data. However, as part of the team, you will have the opportunity to learn lots about other parts of the research process. Most research projects take 3–5 years to complete, from the initial research idea to the writing up and presentation of results. Implementing research into practice comes afterwards, so it is a lengthy process.

As a research midwife, you may have a short-term contract or be on secondment for approximately 12–18 months, depending on the time required for data collection. Your work will be very focused on the research topic, so you need to be interested in the subject area to be able to enjoy the process. Research midwives' clinical experience is very useful for the smooth day to day running of clinical studies. You know and understand midwives and pregnant women. Therefore, you can advise the other researchers on what works and what doesn't work in clinical practice. With time and experience, there will be opportunities to get involved with other aspects of the research process and to gain new skills, as you work on further research studies.

Compared with medical research, midwifery research is relatively young and at present there is no defined career path for research midwives. If you want to pursue a research career you are probably best placed in a large teaching hospital with university links. Health-related bachelor degrees (BA and BSc) can provide a good foundation in, and introduction to research methods and methodology. Should you decide to stay in research, then a course such as an MSc in health service research can provide excellent theoretical and practical experience, relevant to both quantitative and qualitative research methodologies.

It may be your long term goal to undertake a PhD. To achieve this you must find funding, a research study that holds your interest and supervisors that will support you through this long and tough but rewarding journey. Funding opportunities are available for PhDs.

A career in research is pursued for love of the job, not love of money, and the majority of those who undertake research do so because they want to develop and provide a better service and see better outcomes for women and their families in the future. However, this career is not for everybody, and there are many other ways in which midwives can promote research.

Promoting research as a midwife

There are lots of ways in which midwives can promote research in everyday practice, and lots of opportunities to do so. An example is through evidence-based practice — explaining current best practices (determined through research) when giving women choices. These might include recommendations for healthy eating during pregnancy, using water as analgesia in normal labour and breastfeeding for the first six months postnatally.

Midwifery practice is informed by both local hospital guidelines and NICE (National Institute for Health and Clinical Excellence) guidelines. For the highest standard of care to be achieved, practice must be audited against these guidelines, which in turn must be regularly updated in line with the current evidence. Midwives can have involvement in auditing their own practice, and be part of guideline development and updating groups.

Midwives who are keen to keep updated on a specific area may set up journal clubs or attend specific study days — at journal clubs, research papers are critiqued and discussed in line with midwives' current clinical practice and experience, and after attending specific study days, the information gained can then be shared with midwifery colleagues. The internet can also play a role in updating knowledge. Specific groups are accessible to midwives who want to share information, e.g. the 'Birth centres' Yahoo! group and the 'Midwifery research network'.

Gaining further experience as a research midwife

Writing a research protocol

The research protocol is a step by step guide through your study, describing the research process. If you are writing a protocol for the first time, you should seek the help of your hospital's research department, the university and your colleagues on the research team. Writing this document is an important step in starting a research study.

Ethical approval

All research involving pregnant women and/or their babies requires ethical approval. To gain this you must first complete an IRAS (Integrated Research Application

Systems) application. This can be daunting the first time you do it. However, help will be available to you, again from the hospital's research department, the university and your research colleagues. It is very important that your research protocol is complete and ready when you complete an IRAS application.

Funding opportunities

In the current climate funding is tight and well-established research teams have a greater chance of acquiring funds. If you are new to completing grant applications and applying for research funding, you are likely to have greater success applying for smaller amounts and internal funding. Your finance team can support you when completing grant applications so they are well thought through and achievable.

Steering group meetings

Once funding has been secured and the ethical approval process has started, all the relevant stakeholders should be involved, namely: hospital management, academics, clinicians and participant representatives. Their collaboration is vital for getting the study up and running in the clinical area, and to enable regular progress reports throughout the study. The research midwife can contribute to this group by giving feedback of her/his experiences of the study.

Newsletters

Midwives and other clinicians on the ground floor should be kept up to date with the study's progress. They are as much a part of the study as you are and you must keep them engaged. For instance, they will want to know the recruitment figures on a regular basis. A newsletter can publish these figures, which can keep the study at the forefront of their minds. Research usually takes a second place to everyday clinical practice, as it should do. Remember that not all midwives are focused on research or share your interest in research. This newsletter can be written by the research midwife in consultation with the research team/research study manager.

Engaging with participants and midwives

Being a research midwife is all encompassing. You will find that you eat, live and breathe the research study. Your colleagues no longer see you as the midwife colleague you once were, they see you as the research study midwife — for example, the COMET (Comparative Obstetric Mobile Epidural Trial) study midwife (COMET Study Group UK 2001). With this in mind, it is important that you remain approachable to both midwives and participants. They will all have lots of questions and what you can't answer, you should take back to the research team for assistance. This engagement is vital for the smooth running and success of the research study.

Writing research papers and disseminating research results

This is normally done by the principal investigator, in collaboration with other members of the research study team. The research midwife can gain experience from this, for future research publications. Attending study days and presenting the results is an important part of research. Results can be presented orally and/ or be written, as research posters. The research midwife can gain experience at presenting research study results at midwifery study days.

References

Benner P (1984) *From Novice to Expert: Excellence and Power in Clinical Nursing Practice*. Addison-Wesley Publishing Company, California

Bowling A (1997) *Research methods in Health*. Open University, Milton Keynes

Cahill H (1996) A qualitative analysis of student nurses' experiences of mentorship. *J Adv Nurs*. **24(4)**: 791–9

COMET Study Group UK (2001) Effect of low-dose mobile versus traditional epidural techniques on mode of delivery: a randomised controlled trial. *Lancet*. **358(7)**: 19-23

Currie SM (1999) Aspects of the preparation of student midwives for autonomous practice. *Midwifery*. **15**: 283-92

Department of Health. (2009) *Preceptorship Framework for newly registered nurses, midwives and allied health professionals*. DOH, London

Department of Health. (2009) *Education Commissioning For Quality*. DOH, London

Department of Health (2000) *HSC 2000/026: Patient group directions [England only]*. Health & Safety Commission, London

Department of Health (2000) *A Health Service of All the Talents: Developing the NHS workforce. Consultation document on the review of workforce planning*. NHS Executive, Leeds

Donovan P (2008) Confidence in newly qualified midwives. *Br J Midwifery.* **16(8):** 510-4

English National Board for Nursing, Midwifery and Health Visiting (2001) *Placements in focus: Guidance for education in practice for health care professions*. ENB, London

Earnshaw GJ (1995) Mentorship: The students' views. *Nurse Educ Today.* **11:** 225–9

Glen S, Parker P (2003) *Supporting Learning in Practice – A Guide for Practitioners*. Palgrave Macmillan, London

Gray MA, Smith LN (2000) The qualities of an effective mentor from the student nurse's perspective: Findings from a longitudinal qualitative study. *J Adv Nurs.* **32(6):** 1542–9

Haddock J, Bassett C, (1997) Nurses' perceptions of reflective practice. *Nurs Stand.* **11(32):** 39-41.

Hindle T (1998) *Reducing Stress*. Dorling Kindersley, London

Hulatt, I (1995) A Sad Reflection. *Nurs Stand.* **9(20):** 22-3

Jarvis P, Gibson S (Eds) (1997) *The Teacher Practitioner and Mentor in Nursing, Midwifery and Health Visiting and the Social Services. 2nd edn*. Stanley Thornes, Cheltenham

Jarvis P (1992) Reflective Practice and Nursing. *Nurse Educ Today* **12(3):** 174-81

Johns C (2000) *Becoming a Reflective Practitioner*. Wiley-Blackwell, London

Knowles M (1980) *The Modern Practice of Adult Education: From Pedagogy to Androgogy*. Follett, Chicago

Kingscott A (2010) *Supervisors of Midwives: a resource pack*. Birmingham City University

Lloyd Jones M, Walters S, Akehurst R (2001) The implications of contact with the mentor for preregistration nursing and midwifery students. *J Adv Nurs.* **35(2):** 151–60

Locasto LW, Kochanek D (1989) Reality Shock in the Nurse Educator. *J Nurs Educ.* **28(2):** 79–81

Martin V (2000) Managing your time. Part 3. *Nurs Times.* **96(18):** 42

Maslow AH (1943) A Theory of Human Motivation. *Psychology Review.* **50:** 370–96

Mc Candlish R, Bowler U, van Asten H (1998) A randomised controlled trial of care of the perineum during the second stage of normal labour. *Br J Obstet and Gynaecol.* **105(12):** 1262-72

McCarthy, R. (2009) Protecting the perineum: have we been duped by HOOP? *Br J Midwifery.* **17(12):** 779-781

Midwifery 2020 Programme (2010) Midwifery 2020 Delivery Expectations, September www.midwifery2020.org (accessed 5/1/11)

Morton-Cooper A, Palmer A (1993) *Mentoring, Preceptorship and Clinical Supervision: A guide to professional roles in clinical practice 2nd edn.* Wiley-Blackwell, London

Neary M, Phillips R, Davies B (1994) *The Practitioner Teacher: A study in the introduction of mentors in pre-registration Nurse Education Programme in Wales.* School of Education, University of Wales, Cardiff

NHS Careers (2011) Pay for nurses and midwives. www.nhscareers.nhs.uk (accessed 27 February 2011)

Nursing and Midwifery Council (NMC) (2010) *Support for Parents: how supervision and supervisors of midwives can help you.* NMC, London

Nursing and Midwifery Council (NMC) (2009) *Modern supervision in action a practical guide for midwives* NMC, London

Nursing and Midwifery Council (NMC) (2008) *Standards for Pre-registration Midwifery Education.* NMC, London

Nursing and Midwifery Council (NMC) (2008) *Modern Supervision in Action: a practical guide for midwives.* NMC, London

Nursing and Midwifery Council (NMC) (2008) *The Prep Handbook.* NMC, London

Nursing and Midwifery Council (NMC) (2006) *Standards for the Preparation and Practice of Supervisors of Midwives.* NMC, London

Nursing and Midwifery Council (NMC) (2004) *Midwives Rules and Standards.* NMC, London

Nursing and Midwifery Council (NMC) (2002) *Supporting Nurses and Midwives Through Lifelong Learning.* NMC, London

Polit D, Hungler B (1995) *Nursing Research; principles and methods.* Lippincott, Philadelphia

Shepherd S, Doll H, Jenkinson C (1997) Randomised controlled trials cited in Scott C (1999) A description of the roles, activities and skills of clinical nurse specialists in the United States. *Clin Nurse Spec.* **13(4):** 183-90

Smith C, Crowther C, Beilby J (2002) Acupuncture to treat nausea and vomiting in early pregnancy: a randomised controlled trial. *Complement Ther Med.* **10(2):** 78-83

Thomas N (2007) Roles and Responsibilities of the Supervisor of Midwives. In: NMC *Statutory Supervision of Midwives: a resource for midwives and mothers.* MA Healthcare, London.

Chapter 2

Developing as a midwife

- What is involved in continuing professional development?
- How can I develop my professional practice?
- What can my Supervisor of Midwives do for me?
- How can I ensure that I reflect on midwifery practice?
- What will it be like to mentor a student midwife?
- What is involved in teaching a student midwife?

What is involved in continuing professional development?
Claire Agnew/Jacqui Williams

'All midwives will recognise that their learning continues after graduation, they will have access to relevant, timely continuing professional education and will have sufficient time to take part in this education.'
Midwifery 2020 Programme (2010)

As midwives, we are accountable for maintaining high standards of professional practice. The midwifery environment is one of constant change and it is vital that all midwives are able to keep up with the changes. A key role of your Supervisor of Midwives is to encourage your ongoing personal and professional development, promoting lifelong learning (NMC 2009).

The concept of lifelong learning is embraced by post-registration education and practice (Prep), a set of Nursing and Midwifery Council (NMC) standards and guidelines that enable you to demonstrate that you are keeping up to date with developments in professional practice (NMC 2008a). These include keeping a personal professional profile (see Box 2.1) and completing a certain number of hours of continuing professional development (CPD) activities. This is in addition to any of the mandatory training that your Trust asks you to attend.

The Prep handbook is a comprehensive guide to meeting these standards and is available free of charge through the organisation's website (www.nmc-uk.org).

Each year, you will need to do the following to renew your registration:

- Provide a signed Notification of practice (NoP) form and pay a renewal of registration fee.
- The NoP form includes a declaration that you have met the Prep requirements and are of good health and good character.
- Your registration will not be renewed until the NMC has processed your completed and signed form, together with your fee payment.
- In accordance with rule 3 of the Midwives rules and standards (NMC 2004), you must also provide notice of your intention to practise. This is also done annually, by submitting a completed Intention to practise (ItP) form to your named Supervisor of Midwives

Two separate Prep standards must be met in order to maintain registration as a midwife:

- **The Prep (practice) standard** — You must have practised as a midwife for a minimum of 450 hours during the last three years, or have successfully undertaken an approved return to practice course within the last three years.
- **The Prep continuing professional development (CPD) standard** — You must have undertaken and recorded at least 35 hours of learning activity relevant to your midwifery practice during the three years prior to your renewal of registration.
Prep does not have to cost you any money. Furthermore:

- There is no such thing as a Prep-approved CPD activity.
- There is no requirement to collect points or certificates.
- There is no approved format for the personal professional profile.

A way in which you can plan how to meet Prep requirements is through appraisal, or individual performance reviews (Wheeler 2001). This offers a chance to sit down with your manager and plan your career. Your aspirations can be as simple as surviving night shifts — the important thing is that you have the opportunity to discuss your strengths and weaknesses and to develop an action plan for achieving your goals. In the author's experience, new midwives tend to focus on learning practical skills, such as epidural top ups and suturing; it is important that you do not overlook your development in areas such as assertiveness, team working and time management.

Box 2.1 What a professional profile will do for you

- Help you to assess your current standards of practice
- Develop your analytical skills
- Review and evaluate your past experiences
- Demonstrate experiential learning
- Assist with job or course applications

Planning your professional development should include:

- A review of your competence.
- Reflection on how you think you are doing.
- A record of hours spent studying and your learning outcomes.
- Setting learning objectives.
- Developing an action plan.
- Implementing an action plan.
- SWOT Analysis:
  - Strengths e.g. professional manner, easy to get on with, friendly but assertive
  - Weaknesses e.g. can't say no, leave things until the last minute
  - Opportunities e.g. secondment, shadowing other staff, being a mentor
  - Threats e.g. shortage of staff, keeping motivated, over-committing yourself.
- A record of the following:
  - Your name and your appraiser's name, your signatures and the date
  - Your manager's job title
  - The review date
  - Your career aspirations/development pathway.

How can I develop my midwifery practice?
John Fowler/Jacqui Williams

There are many opportunities for professional development. At any one time, those that are available to you will vary depending on:

- Your vision for your career pathway.
- Your strengths and weaknesses.

- The amount of additional time that you are willing and able to invest in your own development.
- The culture of your work setting.

You must take an active role in seeking out and taking these opportunities. Professional development cannot happen in isolation. Your clinical experience will also deepen your knowledge and interpersonal skills. If you are to gain an in-depth knowledge of midwifery practice, you must continue to build on your knowledge base. This will involve developing skills specific to the area that you work in.

You will likely be given the opportunity to rotate around different midwifery areas within your Trust, to consolidate and broaden your practice. Initially, you can expect to be employed as a band 5 but with additional skills' training and assessment, you can become a band 6 by the end of your first year (NHS Careers 2011). Some areas, such as London, may recruit newly qualified midwives straight onto a band 6.

As well as providing evidence of your professional development every six months, each year there will be mandatory updates to your training. These compulsory sessions may focus on skills such as manual handling, cardio-pulmonary resuscitation (both for adults and newborns), fire procedures, child protection, electronic fetal monitoring, the management of obstetric emergencies and record keeping.

Preceptorship

Jacqui Williams

One of the most effective ways of ensuring that you learn and develop with your clinical experience is to enlist the help and advice of somebody more experienced than yourself. In midwifery, support is given during the post-qualification transition phase, during which time you will adjust to your new role and be enabled to develop professionally. However, you must remember that your professional programme will have prepared you to not only be safe and competent but also to be accountable from the point of registration (NMC 2004). There is an expectation that you are ready to undertake the role of midwife, albeit as a novice practitioner (DoH 2009).

Preceptorship will enable you to develop a range of competencies relating to your particular midwifery practice, such as suturing, drug administration and epidural top ups. Importantly, during this period you will both apply and develop the knowledge you have gained in your midwifery undergraduate programme.

The NMC (2006) defines **preceptorship** as:

'...about providing support and guidance enabling new registrants to make the transition from student to accountable practitioner ... to develop confidence as a ...midwife...'

A **preceptor** is defined as:

'a registered practitioner who has been given a formal responsibility to support a newly registered practitioner...'

(DoH 2009a)

During this period, you will be encouraged to grow both in confidence and job satisfaction (DoH 2009a). Your Trust will likely provide a range of learning methods, meaning that your preceptorship can be personalised.

Preceptorship involves the identification of your learning needs and their discussion with a more senior midwife. Each year you will have an individual performance review (IPR) and you should have all the training that you require to meet your needs and the needs your employer. There are many ways in which this can be achieved, including single study days, in-service training, short courses and open learning programmes.

'...skills required for taking on the role of lead carer for women with complex medical and/or obstetric needs is developmental, and competence is to be achieved after initial registration.'

(NMC 2008a)

Should I do a post-registration course?

Nigel Goodrich/John Fowler/Jacqui Williams

The majority of universities that provide undergraduate midwifery training will also have a post-registration degree that is part of the NMC framework. Discuss you career aspirations with your line manager during your IPR, so you can plan for any future courses that you may like to do or even take single courses/modules to develop your knowledge and expertise.

Box 2.2 Example advertisement

MSc/PG Dip/PG Cert — Midwifery Practice

A course designed for midwives who wish to undertake a part-time postgraduate course which prepares them for senior positions in practice, management, research or education.

- Ideal for midwives thinking of careers in management, education and as consultant midwives
- Apply critical reflection and theory to practice
- Implement change in practice as a consequence of study and research
- Partnership teaching and support between the University and employing NHS trust.

Attendance for taught sessions only, three–four hours per week for 10–12 weeks per semester.

Entry requirements

Professional midwifery qualification with evidence of current registration as a midwife with the Nursing and Midwifery Council.

- Employed in the UK as a midwife with an employer willing to provide a clinical mentor during the course, plus either
- An Honours degree (2:2 minimum) in a degree relevant to midwifery and awarded by a British university, or
- Portfolio evidence which demonstrates expertise through publication, change management and/or leadership in midwifery and successful study at level 3 at a British university.

Career opportunities

Completing the MSc Midwifery supports midwives' development in clinical practice and may facilitate career progression to more senior posts within NHS Trusts or within higher education institutions.

This course aims to:

- Facilitate the development of innovative leaders in the midwifery profession who will make a substantial contribution to the development of practice
- Provide theoretical and research modules based firmly on advanced study of practices and challenges which you may face in clinical practice
- Develop inter-professional learning and the exchange of ideas that will enhance your learning across both professional and specific practice boundaries.

You can expect to study from a range of modules, including:

- Research Designs in Health
- Midwifery Theory and Practice
- Dissertation.

This course offers different options as you can also choose to study option modules up to the value of 60 credits from a range available within the Faculty, some of which can be at level 3.

Source: www.dmu.ac.uk

Specialist roles

In order for you to progress in your career, you may contemplate such posts as midwifery specialist, practice development midwife nurse or midwifery lecturer. To apply for these posts, you will normally need at least two years' further experience, including experience of leadership and management, and you will be expected to have commenced or completed an appropriate Master's degree. It is quite probable that future midwife consultants will not only have national reputations of clinical excellence, but also reputations for research and be engaged in or have completed doctorate degree studies.

If this all seems a bit daunting and remote from midwifery care, do not despair — the majority of post-registration midwifery courses are designed to enhance and develop women's care. Not all midwives need to be undertaking post-registration degrees. However, if you want to take a key role in developing women-centred care, then you need to consider how you will acquire the appropriate underpinning skills, knowledge and attitude necessary for developing professional practice.

Working in a research role

Karen Jackson/Jacqui Williams

If you want to undertake research in your area, then you must plan very carefully. Factors to consider are:

* Whose cooperation you will need, both to carry out the project and to change practice on the basis of any findings.
* Any ethical considerations.
* Whether or not you will need any support to undertake the work, e.g. freeing up time, administrative support.

Poorly done research will do nothing to enhance your reputation. It may be appropriate to identify opportunities within midwifery services at this stage of your career, if promoting research is something you are interested in. Many trusts have a research and development directorate, which may be able to offer advice and support, or it might be possible to seek the involvement of a local university. Think about setting up an interest group with like-minded colleagues to share ideas and good practice.

What can my Supervisor of Midwives do for me?

Rowena Doughty/Jacqui Williams

Midwifery Supervision is a statutory mechanism, with the primary aim of protecting the public through the promotion of safe and effective standards of midwifery care (NMC 2008a).

Whatever setting you work in, when you take up your midwifery post, you will be allocated a named Supervisor of Midwives (SoM). You can, however, approach any SoM in your area. A SoM is an experienced midwife who has undergone additional training and education to take on this role. The Local Supervising Authority (LSA) will have appointed her to supervise a number of midwives within its area (NMC 2004, 2006).

From day one, midwives are accountable for their practice; rule 6 of Midwives Rules and Standards (NMC 2004) clearly sets out a midwife's responsibility and sphere of practice. The SoM's role is pivotal in supporting midwives to practice at this level of autonomy (Kingscott 2010).

SoM's have a variety of responsibilities, to:

- Provide professional leadership — to develop evidence-based midwifery practice, with involvement in leading and managing change.
- Monitor local standards of midwifery care.
- Support midwives who are supporting women with their birth plans.
- Verify that the statutory requirements for registration and practice have been met by individual midwives e.g. by processing ItP's (NMC 2008b).
- Investigate any critical incidents or alleged misconduct.
- Provide developmental and supported practice learning packages.
- Provide guidance to individual midwives — be available to discuss their practice, provide guidance to maintain their NMC registration, identify areas for development and training, and provide support.
- Play a part in clinical governance.
- Provide support to women and their families (NMC 2010).
- Engage actively with the maternity services
- Promote birth as a normal physiological process.
- Liaise between educational institutions and practices (Kingscott 2010).

The qualities that you can expect in your SoM are that they are:

- Approachable.
- Committed to woman-centred care.
- A source of professional knowledge and expertise.
- Visionary and inspiring.
- Able to resolve conflict.
- Motivated and thorough.
- Articulate.
- Trustworthy.
- Sympathetic and encouraging.
- Fair and equitable (NMC 2008b).

If midwives feel empowered by their SoM, they are able to empower the women they care for. Therefore, it is important that your relationship with your SoM is a positive one (Thomas 2007).

Key roles of your SoM:

- To meet with you at least annually, to review your practice and identify any training or educational needs.
- To facilitate your professional development.
- To be available to discuss any issues that may arise in practice, such as those following difficult experiences e.g. shoulder dystocia or caring for a woman who has experienced a stillbirth — all discussions will be kept confidential unless action is called for in the interests of safety (NMC 2008h)
- To provide guidance when caring for a woman whose birth plan falls outside accepted care pathways.
- To be available for support and advice to maintain your practice.
- To offer advice on reflective practice.
- To provide support to enable you to achieve your Prep requirements (NMC 2008c).
- To review and audit your record keeping.
- To receive and process your Intention to Practice (ItP) form each year.

Every area has a process in place that enables 24-hour access to a SoM (i.e. in an emergency), although this won't necessarily be your named SoM. If you are involved in a serious incident at work, midwifery supervision will support you in various ways:

- A SoM may undertake a formal investigation of the incident and prepare a supervisory report for the Local Supervising Authority Midwifery Officer (LSAMO)
- If a period of supervised practice is recommended then a SoM, with support from a midwifery educationalist, will develop a package of learning outcomes; the SoM will also monitor progress during this period (NMC 2007)
- The midwife's SoM will also provide support during the investigation and during any period of supervised practice, if appropriate.

A SoM will also identify any midwife who needs additional support and in some cases a period of developmental practice may be created to enhance their skills and knowledge (NMC 2006). As the NMC's 'Modern Supervision in Action: a practical guide for midwives' (NMC 2008b) encourages, you should ask yourself the following questions:

- How can I contact my named supervisor?
- How often do I seek out my named supervisor?
- Do I make the most of supervision?
- Would I consider becoming a Supervisor of Midwives?

How can I ensure that I reflect on midwifery practice?
Claire Agnew/Jacqui Williams

Learning is not achieved solely through having experiences or by attending study days. It is a result of thought and consideration — reflecting on what your experiences actually mean to you. The ability to effectively reflect is fundamental to the development of professional practice (Andrews 1996). Reflection is also an important part of reviewing your strengths and weaknesses and identifying areas that need developing. It means thinking about an event, analysing what occurred, what your thoughts and feelings about the event were, and identifying what you did well and what you might learn from it.

Situations that you should reflect upon include:

- Something you enjoyed or that went well.
- Something you found difficult to deal with.
- A situation where things went wrong.
- A crisis or a midwifery emergency.
- Something you do every day in your midwifery practice.
- Something you rarely do.
      (adapted from Jarvis 1992, Haddock and Bassett 1997; Johns 2000)

A reminder of how to reflect

Although how you choose to reflect on your practice and experiences is a personal decision, it is recommended that you choose a model that will guide you through the stages of reflective learning. Sharing your reflections with someone you feel comfortable with may provide another way of looking at the situation.

Gibbs' reflective cycle (1988; Figure 2.3) provides a simple approach to reflection and Figure 2.4 shows a framework that you may find useful. It is important that you see reflection as a useful tool for developing your midwifery practice and not just an academic exercise that you had to do during your midwifery programme. Record your reflections in your professional portfolio.

What will it be like to be a mentor to a student midwife?
Karen Mee

There is currently a much greater emphasis on student support in the clinical setting than used to be the case (DoH 2000a, 2000b; English National Board for Nursing, Midwifery and Health Visiting 2001). A recent review has sought to offer clarity and direction regarding the support of learners in practice settings,

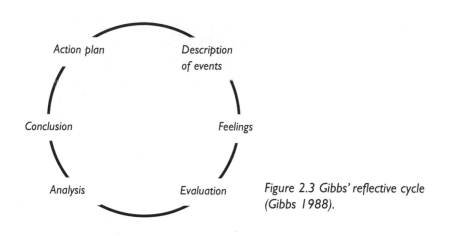

Figure 2.3 Gibbs' reflective cycle (Gibbs 1988).

Description (what happened?)
Feelings (what were you thinking and feeling?) and evaluation (what was good and bad about the experience?)
Analysis (what sense can you make of the situation?)
Conclusion (what else could you have done?)
Action plan and learning outcome
Signature

Figure 2.4. Framework for reflection using the reflective cycle.

and work has been done to develop and implement a range of standards and quality assurance processes for clinical education (DoH 2009b). Nursing and midwifery mentorship has also recently been subject to a professional body review. The NMC (2008) has been instrumental in developing clear standards for mentors supporting students in the practice setting, which have replaced previous standards (NMC 2008).

A variety of new clinical roles have developed, which can support the education of the student midwife or more junior midwife undertaking additional post-registration professional development and further education. In some areas, the contribution of senior students supporting more junior students has been officially recognised through 'buddying' systems.

However, there is little doubt that the most important people in the everyday practice-based lives of midwifery students are the qualified midwives. They are there, all the time, fulfilling the role to which the students aspire. Midwives are the most likely to be allocated the task of 'looking after' students, so:

- How do you do it?
- What skills do you need?
- How can those skills be developed?

First, it may be helpful to clear up a few common misconceptions and give some working definitions of the different types of assessors within the clinical area.

Mentors/Sign-off mentors

Generally speaking, midwifery students can and will be supervised by a whole range of professionals throughout the course of their studies, including nurses, health visitors, social workers, operating department practitioners and doctors. All of these people, provided that they understand the nature, type and content of the midwifery curriculum, can make an important contribution to the learning experience of the student. While those professionals who are not registered midwives can also contribute to student assessment (by providing feedback, for instance), any formal assessment of the achievement of midwifery competence and proficiency must be completed by a registered midwife who has undergone further preparation and training. The NMC has defined two main formal roles for nurses and midwives who support and assess students — mentor and sign-off mentor.

What is a mentor?

A NMC mentor is a registrant who has successfully completed an NMC-approved mentor preparation programme, acquiring the knowledge, skills and competence required to meet their defined criteria.

What is a sign-off mentor?

A sign-off mentor meets the standard mentoring criteria in full, together with additional NMC criteria that are necessary for achieving sign-off status (NMC 2008). The NMC (2008) has made a clear distinction between the roles of mentor and sign-off mentor and has directed that only mentors with sign-off status are eligible to assess the competence of students on NMC-approved pre-registration midwifery education programmes. Sign-off mentors are responsible for confirming that the required proficiencies for entry to the register have been achieved (NMC 2008).

What preparation will I receive to become a mentor?

Since 2001, the NMC has given mentor preparation courses much more definition and clarity (NMC 2004, 2008). The local placement provider holds a register of mentors who have undergone further preparation courses, which is subject to regular updating and CPD/registration, enabling students to be placed with appropriately-trained mentors. Midwives who are not on this register now have to undertake new courses to meet the additional criteria for sign-off mentor status, before becoming official named mentors.

To learn more about the course in your area, you must refer to local information. However, some of the standard criteria for sign-off mentors include:

- Being registered in the same part or sub-part of the register as the student who is being assessed.
- Having developed their own knowledge, skills and competence beyond registration (must have been registered for at least a year).
- Having clinical currency and capability in the field in which the student is being assessed (NMC 2008).
- Successful completion of an NMC-approved mentor preparation programme.
- Confirmation of sign-off proficiency (being supervised on at least three occasions for by an existing sign-off mentor during the programme) (NMC 2008).
- Being able to make judgements about the competence and proficiency of NMC students and being accountable for their decisions (NMC 2008).

- Having an in-depth understanding of their accountability to the NMC for the decision to pass or fail a student when assessing their proficiency at the end of the programme (NMC 2008).

Although widely welcomed, these changes have created challenges for all stakeholders in midwifery education. Perhaps the most significant challenge is that in many areas, in the short term, the new courses simply cannot prepare enough new sign off mentors to meet demands. This has led to the development of distance/open learning courses.

With the introduction of associate/secondary mentors and concepts such as team mentoring, the contributions of those who are not NMC-recognised mentors (professional midwives and others) has been acknowledged. There are many professionals who have undergone some basic preparation for the role, who are able to supervise midwifery students with confidence and who contribute to assessment by providing feedback to both the student and the named mentor. Nonetheless, it is the named mentor who has undergone formal preparation and who should complete the formal assessment.

What competencies will I need to be a mentor?

By now you may be wondering what the mentoring role involves, asking yourself questions such as, 'what am I responsible for?' and 'what skills and competencies will I need?'

The NMC (2008) has designed a developmental framework for mentors, which answers these questions by outlining the activities that underpin effective mentoring. There are eight domains or competencies:

- Establishing effective working relationships.
- Facilitation of learning.
- Assessment and accountability.
- Evaluation of learning.
- Creating an environment for learning.
- Context of practice.
- Evidence-based practice.
- Leadership.

What is involved in mentoring a student?

We know that a mentor is a person who facilitates learning and supervises and assesses students while they are gaining practical experience, but what does this mean in real terms? Lloyd Jones *et al* (2001) add 'general support' and 'acting as a role model' to the list of competencies, and make the point that the term 'mentor' is misleading, considering the short duration of placements. Neary *et al* (1994) describe a good mentor as someone who possesses appropriate professional attributes, knowledge, good communication skills, and who has the motivation to teach and support students.

A distinction can be made between formal and informal mentoring. While statutory bodies are only concerned with the former, informal mentoring's importance should nevertheless be professionally acknowledged. If we accept this and see mentoring as a positive endeavour, we might then add other dimensions to the role, such as 'knowledgeable friend', 'helper', 'advocate', 'challenger' (Earnshaw 1995; Cahill 1996), 'coach', 'counsellor', 'guide' (Morton-Cooper and Palmer 1993) and perhaps even 'confidante' (Glen and Parker 2003).

Creating a relationship with your student

While it may seem obvious that the quality of the student-mentor relationship is important for successful mentoring, Jarvis and Gibson (1997) suggest that the relationship does not have to be of a particular type, arguing that it can be as informal or as formal as the different types of mentoring themselves. They conclude that mentorship should provide the opportunity to create a dialogue between student and mentor, where both feel needed. However, both parties must feel confident and comfortable with each other for this to be successful.

One of the most important aspects of building the relationship and making mentorship work is regular contact (Lloyd Jones *et al* 2001). The most obvious way to achieve this is to try to work together as frequently as possible, especially when the mentor is involved in giving care. This approach has three benefits:

- It allows the student to learn by observing first hand.
- It allows the mentor to demonstrate sufficient confidence in their own skills, that they are happy to be scrutinised.
- It can encourage the development of trust and respect between mentor and student, as they begin to see each other as colleagues.

Opportunities to work together are made easier considering that students are now exposed to 24/7 care from early on in their studies — with appropriate negotiation, it should be possible to go some way towards having matching duty schedules. This also helps to fulfil the statutory obligation that the mentor is required to:

'...use knowledge of the student's stage of learning to select appropriate opportunities to meet individual needs.'

(NMC 2008)

However, with such focus on assessment, signing off and the implicit power dynamic, it can be hard for students to be honest, open and to admit to shortfalls in knowledge.

Spouse (1996) has suggested that basic methods, such as the mentor initiating social interactions, can optimise this relationship. Having a chat, taking a personal interest, and sharing personal feelings and experiences can show warmth, promote trust and enable students to see their mentors as real people.

Gray and Smith (2000) summarised this neatly when they concluded that having a good mentor usually coincides with having a good placement. Rather more anecdotally, it is worth noting that I regularly have cause to ask students about their practical experiences and specifically about what they believe constitutes a good practice placement — answers consistently come back along the following lines:

- 'They actually knew that I existed and were expecting me.'
- 'My mentor made me feel welcome and took an interest in me.'
- 'They seemed to like having students and wanted to teach me.'
- 'They were always willing to ask me questions, and help me find out the answers if I didn't know.'
- 'They didn't mind me asking questions or feel threatened by me asking them.'
- 'They really know their stuff on that ward.'
- 'They didn't just leave the students to fend for themselves.'
- 'Even when they were busy, they didn't make me feel like a nuisance.'

Even in a climate of staff shortages and with difficulties filling vacancies, such discussions with students often end with:

'I'd love to go back there to work as a qualified midwife.'

To summarise this section, the suggestions that arose from Gray and Smith's study into the qualities of a good mentor (2000) make a helpful checklist:

- Enthusiastic.
- Friendly.
- Approachable.
- Patient and understanding.
- Good sense of humour.
- Good role model.
- Professional and organised.
- Caring and self-confident.
- Good communicator.
- Knowledgeable about the student's course.
- Has realistic expectations of (plus confidence and trust in) the student's abilities.
- Provides regular feedback.
- Involves the student in activities.
- Spends time with the student.
- Shows a genuine interest in the student.
- Is willing and able to gradually reduce the level of direct supervision.

No-one said that being a mentor was going to be easy.

Giving feedback

Formal assessment of students will be examined at a later stage in this chapter. Formative assessment is usually defined as the provision of feedback on a student's progress, which is not used to make specific judgements about passing or failing. A typical example of a formative assessment might be:

> *'When you cared for Amira in labour yesterday I noticed you paid particular attention to trying to build up a rapport and gained her informed consent for any procedures. Next time also consider how you involve her partner more in her care.'*

Generally speaking, we find it easier to give praise than to criticise, yet ironically students often report that the only feedback they get is about their failings — often too late for them to be able to do anything about. Two golden rules about giving feedback might be seen to emerge from this last statement:

- Do not hesitate to provide positive feedback and praise on a student's performance, i.e. do not rely on the maxim 'no news is good news'.
- If things are not going well, then make sure the student knows as early as possible.

The objective here is to ensure that the student has as much time as possible to put matters right and, hopefully, avoid failing an assessment. Incidentally, you might consider it good practice to let the module leader at the university know at the same time so that s/he can support the student (and you) early on as well.

Students want and need feedback on both their strengths and weaknesses. They cannot engage in effective reflection and thereby refocus their learning if they do not know how well they are doing. So long as the relationship is built on mutual trust and respect (as discussed earlier), students value constructive criticism about their knowledge, skills and attitudes. The proviso is that any such feedback should be discreet and take place away from the woman (Spouse 1996) and other members of staff.

Having made this last point, it is only fair to point out that as the mentor of the student, you will receive feedback from other members of the team (with whom the student may have worked while you were not there).

It will take skill and courage to talk to the student about 'second hand' issues and concerns, while ensuring that the student remains convinced of the professional value of other supervisors reporting their opinions to you. Ideally, only the named midwife should provide feedback to the student. However, it is acknowledged that sometimes feedback cannot wait and has to be given immediately.

What is involved in teaching a student?
Paul Pleasance/Deborah Dowsett/Jacqui Williams

Of all the aspects of the mentor role, perhaps the most valued by students is the teaching component — this is a theme that recurs throughout the research literature (Spouse 1996, Andrews and Chilton 2000, Gray and Smith 2000). Students realise that there is much more to teaching than being taken away from the ward environment — perhaps to a day room or an empty side ward — and sitting down to receive a lecture from one of the team. That is not to say that there is not a place for this on occasion — there undoubtedly is, and students enjoy it.

Some of the principles outlined in subsequent sections might apply equally to formal and informal teaching opportunities. It is clear that formal lecturing is not the only way of teaching learners.

Setting learning outcomes

In the world of education, the relative merits of 'objectives' and 'outcomes' have been debated for many years. It can be argued that the term 'outcomes' is more helpful, as the focus is on what should be learned ('student-centred') rather than on what should be taught ('teacher-centred') or on what students should be able to do ('behavioural objectives') — but this is all just semantics. The important thing is to identify students' learning needs and the learning opportunities provided by the practice placement environment.

Your first question might be, 'what is the student here for?' The simplest answer is 'to learn how to be a midwife — the practical side of the job'. After all, you might argue that the university provides the theory; but that would undervalue your expertise as a qualified midwife/mentor. You do not just know about the practical side of midwifery, you are an expert in its theoretical underpinnings. So, have the confidence to see yourself as an expert (this is not the same as suggesting that you know everything) — teaching a student is about being able to share this expertise, both the theory and the practice.

It is a reasonable expectation that students should be able to specify what they want and/or need to learn while allocated to your area — if not, you might send them away to come back the next day, having identified some of their intentions. The university will have provided the students with some guidance regarding what they might expect to get out of the experience. It is also a reasonable expectation that you will be able to identify both the general and unique learning opportunities that your practice environment can provide. If not, sit down with your colleagues and identify them. You can then include your conclusions in the induction pack that you give all students on their first day in your practice setting.

When you have identified the student's learning needs and the learning opportunities that the placement offers, you can then identify learning outcomes, which will be a marriage of the two. Of course, you must also consider a range of other issues to set the context of this exercise, for example:

- How long is the student to be placed with you?
- What stage of the course is the student at?

- Are you planning an individual teaching session, a day of supervised practice, or the whole allocation?
- What learning outcomes have already been set that the student has to meet?

The main value of identifying anticipated learning outcomes is that it ensures that all parties (yourself, the student and the other members of the midwifery team) know and understand the purpose of the allocation. Learning outcomes can also be used to show everybody what they can contribute to the student's learning.

In summary:

- Learning outcomes should reflect the matches between what the student wants and/or needs to know, and what learning opportunities are presented by the practice environment.
- Consider how the student is best supported to meet the required learning outcomes.

The learning environment

Most students do want to learn. Although the way they present themselves and voice their desires may be different from what we expect, the majority are still highly vocationally oriented and want to learn all the things necessary for them to become good professional midwives. This goes a long way towards ensuring solid, intrinsic motivation to learn, as opposed to the extrinsic types of motivation borne only out of such things as obligation, compulsion and fear of failure.

The classic work of Maslow (1943) suggests that before effective new learning can take place, all other more basic needs need to be addressed. Despite its age, Maslow's hierarchy of needs still provides a useful template for assessment of the learning environment, and it reminds teachers of the necessary considerations for creating a setting in which optimal learning can occur. Any person who wants to teach in a practice setting should be able to offer the following:

- A welcoming atmosphere.
- High quality, evidence-based care.
- Repeated opportunities to practise skills under supervision.
- A willingness to ask and answer questions.
- A willingness to repeat explanations — once is rarely enough.
- Skills, competence and confidence — teachers are role models.
- Clear and effective links with the educational institution.
- Recognition of students' learning needs.

- Effective team leadership and good staff relations.
- Time dedicated to teaching, including the use of 'quiet time'.

It is no coincidence that there is much common ground between the above list and the characteristics of good mentors and good placements as discussed earlier. However, one of the most significant obstacles to professional learning, as reported by students, is that they are sometimes unsure of what they need to know. If students do not know what they need to know, it is unlikely that they will be able to identify and utilise learning opportunities effectively. It sometimes happens, then, that those students end up repeating the same activities over and over again, and fail to move on to develop other skills and knowledge.

'Concepts of confidence and competence may be linked but they are not synomous. Increased levels of confidence are not in direct proportion to increasing competence although decreasing confidence may be linked to a reduction in skilled performance and the need and request for more direct supervision.'

(Donovan 2008)

Good mentoring can promote confidence in students and together with constructive criticism, praise is key to this (Currie 1999). Students need feedback on their progress in developing skills and making decisions so that their confidence can also grow (Donovan 2008).

Learning resources

The learning environment is, or should be, an important learning resource. Knowles (1980) proposed that adults need to feel accepted, respected and supported in their learning and be able to express their feelings without being ridiculed.

In your area, there are essentially three learning resources open to the student:

- You (the student's mentor).
- Other members of the multidisciplinary team.
- The practice environment itself — specifically, the women who are there to be cared for.

This last point raises some ethical concerns, as it infers that women are being used for professional purposes, which of course they are. Many of these concerns are effectively eliminated, given that students are supervised in practice but theoretically, patients can decline to have students of any kind involved in their care.

It is the mentor's role to plan and coordinate the student's experience, to ensure the best opportunities and to capitalise on what each of the three learning resources can offer — if there appear to be gaps in the range of available opportunities then the mentor can often create and utilise alternatives. This could mean, for example, organising activities so that the student can:

- Spend some of, or the whole of a shift in a different area, such as on the maternity assessment unit.
- Work with specific colleagues who have specific expertise e.g. a Diabetes Specialist Midwife.
- Observe techniques or procedures e.g. fetal blood sampling, amniocentesis.
- Escort a woman e.g. to the neonatal unit.
- Follow the woman's journey.
- Follow up a new practice experience with some theory input.
- Obtain evidence to support a practice intervention.

Although often shunned by midwives in their search for professional respectability, students can also learn from different cultural practices (e.g. care during labour) and from the history of midwifery (e.g. changes in breast feeding practices). Practitioners needn't fear this kind of knowledge, especially where cultures have embraced the concept of evidence. Not everything can be learned from books or in a classroom, and the professional practice-based mentor is uniquely placed to help the student to learn.

Approaches to teaching

It is beyond the scope of this chapter to provide a training programme that teaches mentors how to teach their students. However, it can provide some pointers that might form a basis for reflection, from which the mentor may start to develop a personal philosophy of how they should approach teaching. For instance, in the past 20 or so years, it has become popular for educationalists to debate the relative merits of pedagogy (traditionally used to describe the art and science of teaching, which now tends to be reserved for the teaching of children) and androgogy (usually reserved to describe the art and science of teaching adults). Knowles

(1973) was one of the first to describe such a theory, and concluded that adults learn best when:

- Learning is self directed.
- Learning is related to their past experience.
- Whatever is to be learned is relevant to their everyday life.
- Learning material is of a problem-solving nature.

One might argue that midwives and nurses (and probably their university departments) are more comfortable with an approach that tends towards pedagogy, especially when compared with other professional student groups. If it seems appropriate, you shouldn't be afraid to take this approach. The important thing is to get to know the student, so that you both feel comfortable enough to allow flexibility in the way that things are taught — and learned.

Finally, whichever approach you take, the emphasis needs to be upon 'learning'. You can teach and facilitate all day but if the student is not learning, it is a complete waste of time.

What is involved in assessing a student?
Paul Pleasance/Deborah Dowsett/Jacqui Williams

The good part of student assessment is that it acknowledges achievements and marks the progression towards registration. The bad part is that students sometimes fail. We will look at this a little later.

Formative assessment

This was defined earlier as the provision of feedback on a student's progress, which is not used to make specific judgements about the student passing or failing.

Summative assessment

Conversely, this is the pass/fail judgment, which is used to decide whether or not a student can progress on their course and, ultimately, qualify as a midwife.

Characteristics of assessment

In collaboration with colleagues from the service, each university midwifery department is required to formulate assessment tools for the theory and practice components of the course. There is a shared commitment to ensuring that all assessments are:

- **Valid** — they assess what they are supposed to assess.
- **Reliable** — that the outcomes of assessment are consistent, irrespective of when assessment takes place and who completes it.
- **Discriminating** — that a 'good' student will pass and a 'bad' student will fail.
- **Practical** — demands on the assessor, in terms of resources such as time and money, must be reasonable.

Although it is not uncommon for practice-based staff to be involved in theory-based assessments, it is much more likely for them to be involved in the assessment of practice-based competence.

When preparing to undertake a mentoring role — and also as a part of annual updating — you should ensure that you are familiar with the nature, type, content and use of assessment documents at your area's university. If you are uncertain of any specific requirements, then contact a member of the faculty for guidance before you need their help (see earlier section on liaising with the university).

What is assessed?

Although different universities' assessments vary, you will find certain things in common. For example, all assessment documents will monitor and record the student's ongoing achievement in:

- Practical skills.
- Intellectual skills.
- Interpersonal skills, including:
  - Ability to work within a team
  - Ability to relate to women and their partners.
- Integration of theory and practice.
- Professionalism/professional conduct.

Pitfalls in assessment

The onus is on the mentor to ensure that assessments are as fair and objective as possible. An advantage of team mentoring is that this responsibility can be shared — no single mentor will be able to work with the student for all of the time that she or he is on duty, so the wise mentor will seek the feedback of other team members, perhaps associate or secondary mentors (see earlier). However, it is the mentor who ultimately decides whether or not the student has achieved all the learning outcomes.

It is worth considering some of the common pitfalls of assessment that the mentor will have to avoid:

- **First impressions** — where the first impression of an individual can distort later perceptions, e.g. if the student is late on the first day, however genuine their reason, staff may make wrong assumptions about other aspects of performance.
- **Halo effect** — where a feature or characteristic exhibited by the student (good or bad) influences or inhibits later observations, e.g. sporting prowess, physical characteristics.
- **Stereotyping** — the subconscious classification of people using assumptions we have 'learned' in the past. Most of us have to make conscious efforts not to make generalised and inappropriate assumptions about groups of people. Reflect for a minute on how the general public tends to characterise midwives.
- **Recency effect** — where our overall view of a person is coloured by our most recent interactions with them. If a nurse performs badly today, we may overlook the fact that she or he performed well on every preceding day, and that there may be a reason for today's poor performance.
- **Interpersonal attraction** — we are not talking lust here! Simply put, if somebody appeals to you, whether physically or emotionally, or if they seem to like you, then your objectivity can be compromised and you may view aspects of their work more favourably. Of course, the opposite can be equally true.
- **Self-fulfilling prophecy** — it seems that, ultimately, people tend to behave how others expect them to. This is perhaps most commonly seen in children, but many of us also experience it in adult life. We do well if we are expected to do well and badly if we are expected to do badly.

Purposes of assessment

Student assessment is a heavy responsibility. This is not diminished when we consider the reasons for performing an assessment in the first place:

- To provide the student with feedback on their progress.
- To motivate the student to achieve outcomes.
- To indicate the effectiveness of instruction.
- To indicate the effectiveness of the curriculum.

While these reasons are usually fairly easy to cope with and are unlikely to cause too much stress, it should be noted that where a student fails to achieve, the 'teacher' (whether university- or practice-based) must investigate the cause and ensure that poor performance is not a reflection of inadequate student support.

What happens if a student is failing?

The next two reasons for assessment can potentially cause a degree of anxiety, as so much depends on them. They are:

- To indicate the suitability of the student to be registered to the statutory body.
- To safeguard standards of midwifery care and the health and wellbeing of the public by maintaining a satisfactory level of fitness to practice in future practitioners.

These are not responsibilities that can be taken lightly. Not every student is suitable for registration or fit to practice, which begs the question — what happens if a student fails? This is a difficult decision to make, which can be uncomfortable and unpleasant. However, there are times when failing the student is the only option.

Remember that assessment is a shared activity between you and the university (and the student) so it is important that you not feel alone. If you have any doubts that your student will succeed, then make sure to discuss your concerns with appropriate university staff as soon as possible — do not just keep them among your colleagues in the placement area. This leads to one of the golden rules of assessment: failure should not come as a surprise to anybody — not the student, not the other members of the ward team, and not the university.

As a part of ongoing mentoring, a failure to make satisfactory progress must be highlighted as early as possible, so that you and the student can sit down together and draw up an action plan (with input from a member of the university module team). This should be designed to help the student overcome their weaknesses and achieve their objectives (i.e. it will help them pass).

If and when, having tried everything in your power, you do have to fail your student, there will be active university involvement. Do not be alarmed or surprised by this — it is not a criticism of you or of your decision, and it should certainly not be interpreted as a pressure to pass this student, or future students. The midwifery programme leader/module leader needs to know the circumstances and must be aware of the full picture if she or he is to present and support your recommendation to the Assessment Board with confidence and authority.

The discussion of actions to take when failing a student may seem a rather negative note on which to conclude a consideration of student support. Thankfully, it is very much the exception rather than the rule — the majority of students do make the grade, so long as they are given clear guidance on what is expected of them. On a more positive note, general feedback within the author's area of work suggests that mentors feel empowered in the role, and enthused by the opportunity they have to make such a vital contribution to midwives' education and training. Mentors, sign-off mentors and practice teachers all have important roles and enhance student learning at every level. They are role models, assessors, they have socialisation roles and they provide quality teaching in the clinical environment. They see this as an investment in their own future and a chance to positively influence the caring and professional ability not only of their students but for the profession as a whole.

Liaising with the university

It is increasingly accepted that midwifery education is shared between the university and the practice environment — that students spend 50% of their time in practice is no longer just considered to be a university requirement. Perhaps more importantly, it is no longer perceived that the university 'does the theory side' and the clinical areas 'do the practice side'. Sharing ownership of midwives' education and training has increased teamwork between the two, which has led to a better understanding of each other's respective needs — a state of affairs that we all want to encourage.

However, it can still be confusing to know who you should contact at the university and when. Some universities prefer the first point of contact be the personal tutor, although others suggest that it should be the module leader or the programme leader. If the relevant names and telephone numbers are not on the assessment document/module guide (that the student should have presented to you) then ask the student to give you details, before there is any need for them. Ultimately, if you have any concerns about a student (or if you want to say how wonderful she or he is) then it really does not matter who you contact at the university, but be prepared to be referred on to the 'right person'. Please do not let this put you off. It is important that lines of communication remain open between the university and the clinical midwives who are supporting the student in practice.

You should remember that a variety of people will be able to deal with many of your queries. Practice placement coordinators, lecturer/practitioners and allocations officers can all be useful contacts, and in many university midwifery departments it is common for specific lecturers to be associated with individual directorates or units. It is worth finding out who your 'link lecturer' is and making use of her or him. You should also find out if there is a midwife in your area who has been identified as 'lead' for student issues — practice areas will often have one. The important thing is to ensure that you familiarise yourself with the existing roles, communication pathways and processes used by those working in partnership across your local organisations, who support mentors in their day to day practice.

References

Benner P (1984) *From Novice to Expert: Excellence and Power in Clinical Nursing Practice*. Addison-Wesley Publishing Company, California

Bowling A (1997) *Research methods in Health.* Open University, Milton Keynes

Cahill H (1996) A qualitative analysis of student nurses' experiences of mentorship. *J Adv Nurs.* **24(4)**: 791–9

COMET Study Group UK (2001) Effect of low-dose mobile versus traditional epidural techniques on mode of delivery: a randomised controlled trial. *Lancet.* **358(7):** 19-23

Currie SM (1999) Aspects of the preparation of student midwives for autonomous practice. *Midwifery.* **15:** 283-92

Department of Health. (2009a) *Preceptorship Framework for newly registered nurses, midwives and allied health professionals.* DOH, London

Department of Health. (2009b) *Education Commissioning For Quality.* DOH, London

Department of Health (2000a) *HSC 2000/026: Patient group directions [England only].* Health & Safety Commission, London

Department of Health (2000b) *A Health Service of All the Talents: Developing the NHS workforce. Consultation document on the review of workforce planning.* NHS Executive, Leeds

Donovan P (2008) Confidence in newly qualified midwives. *Br J Midwifery.* **16(8):** 510-4

English National Board for Nursing, Midwifery and Health Visiting (2001) *Placements in focus: Guidance for education in practice for health care professions.* ENB, London

Earnshaw GJ (1995) Mentorship: The students' views. *Nurse Educ Today.* **11:** 225–9

Glen S, Parker P (2003) *Supporting Learning in Practice – A Guide for Practitioners.* Palgrave Macmillan, London

Gray MA, Smith LN (2000) The qualities of an effective mentor from the student nurse's perspective: Findings from a longitudinal qualitative study. *J Adv Nurs.* **32(6):** 1542–9

Haddock J, Bassett C, (1997) Nurses' perceptions of reflective practice. *Nurs Stand.* **11(32):** 39-41.

Hindle T (1998) *Reducing Stress.* Dorling Kindersley, London

Hulatt, I (1995) A Sad Reflection. *Nurs Stand.* **9(20):** 22-3

Jarvis P, Gibson S (Eds) (1997) *The Teacher Practitioner and Mentor in Nursing, Midwifery and Health Visiting and the Social Services. 2nd edn.* Stanley Thornes, Cheltenham

Jarvis P (1992) Reflective Practice and Nursing. *Nurse Educ Today* **12(3):** 174–81

Johns C (2000) *Becoming a Reflective Practitioner.* Wiley-Blackwell, London

Knowles M (1980) *The Modern Practice of Adult Education: From Pedagogy to Androgogy.* Follett, Chicago

Kingscott A (2010) *Supervisors of Midwives: a resource pack.* Birmingham City University

Lloyd Jones M, Walters S, Akehurst R (2001) The implications of contact with the mentor for preregistration nursing and midwifery students. *J Adv Nurs.* **35(2):** 151–60

Locasto LW, Kochanek D (1989) Reality Shock in the Nurse Educator. *J Nurs Educ.* **28(2):** 79–81

Martin V (2000) Managing your time. Part 3. *Nurs Times.* **96(18):** 42

Maslow AH (1943) A Theory of Human Motivation. *Psychology Review.* **50:** 370–96

Mc Candlish R, Bowler U, van Asten H (1998) A randomised controlled trial of care of the perineum during the second stage of normal labour. *Br J Obstet and Gynaecol.* **105(12):** 1262-72

McCarthy, R. (2009) Protecting the perineum: have we been duped by HOOP? *Br J Midwifery.* **17(12):** 779-781

Midwifery 2020 Programme (2010) Midwifery 2020 Delivery Expectations, September www.midwifery2020.org (accessed 5/1/11)

Morton-Cooper A, Palmer A (1993) *Mentoring, Preceptorship and Clinical Supervision: A guide to professional roles in clinical practice 2nd edn.* Wiley-Blackwell, London

Neary M, Phillips R, Davies B (1994) *The Practitioner Teacher: A study in the introduction of mentors in pre-registration Nurse Education Programme in Wales.* School of Education, University of Wales, Cardiff

NHS Carcers (2011) Pay for nurses and midwives. www.nhscareers.nhs.uk (accessed 27 February 2011)

Nursing and Midwifery Council (NMC) (2010) *Support for Parents: how supervision and supervisors of midwives can help you.* NMC, London

Nursing and Midwifery Council (NMC) (2009) *Modern supervision in action a practical guide for midwives.* NMC, London

Nursing and Midwifery Council (NMC) (2008a) *Standards for Pre-registration Midwifery Education,* NMC, London

Nursing and Midwifery Council (NMC) (2008b) *Modern Supervision in Action. a practical guide for midwives.* NMC, London

Nursing and Midwifery Council (NMC) (2008c) *The Prep Handbook.* NMC, London

Nursing and Midwifery Council (NMC) (2006) *Standards for the Preparation and Practice of Supervisors of Midwives.* NMC, London

Nursing and Midwifery Council (NMC) (2004) *Midwives Rules and Standards.* NMC, London

Nursing and Midwifery Council (NMC) (2002) *Supporting Nurses and Midwives Through Lifelong Learning.* NMC, London

Polit D, Hungler B (1995) *Nursing Research; principles and methods.* Lippincott, Philadelphia

Shepherd S, Doll H, Jenkinson C (1997) Randomised controlled trials cited in Scott C (1999) A description of the roles, activities and skills of clinical nurse specialists in the United States. *Clin Nurse Spec.* **13(4):** 183-90

Smith C, Crowther C, Beilby J (2002) Acupuncture to treat nausea and vomiting in early pregnancy: a randomised controlled trial. *Complement Ther Med.* **10(2):** 78-83

Thomas N (2007) Roles and Responsibilities of the Supervisor of Midwives. In: NMC *Statutory Supervision of Midwives: a resource for midwives and mothers.* MA Healthcare, London.

Chapter 3

Promoting normality

'Midwifery Education will be rooted in normality whilst preparing midwives to care for all women including those with complex medical, obstetric and social needs. It will prepare and develop midwives to be skilled and safe, empathetic and trustworthy with increased emphasis on the principles of autonomy and accountability with multidisciplinary and multi-agency teams'

Midwifery 2020 programme (2010)

- **Why do we need to define normality?**
- **What are the signs of normal progress in labour?**
- **How can I improve my communication with women in labour?**
- **How should I monitor the fetal heart in low risk labours?**
- **What do I need to consider about food and fluids for women in labour**
- **What positions can promote normality in labour?**
- **What do I need to consider when using water in normal labour?**
- **Is music useful in for women in labour?**

Why do we need to define normality?

Sue Nyombi/Jacqui Williams

It could be argued that in the technological age, natural birth is no longer the norm. In consultant units up and down the UK, women give birth lying in a semi-recumbent position on hard delivery beds, are refused nourishment and rely on pharmaceutical pain relief — this is often defined as 'normal labour'.

In her book 'Normal Childbirth' (2008) Soo Downe speaks of the paradox of midwifery — that it claims to be the guardian of normality, yet it encourages the use of technical procedures during labour. Consider the following:

- All consultant units have an established epidural service and if necessary, several women can have epidurals sited at any one time.

- Many units house just one birthing pool, which is only accessible if it is working, if a willing and competent midwife is available, if it is not too busy and if the woman requests it.
- The woman who is mobile during labour, who eats and drinks, gives birth in an upright position and has a physiological third stage is now so rare as to be termed 'abnormal'.
- In everyday practice, amniotomy and episiotomy are common interventions, often carried out by midwives during so-called 'normal' labours. Moreover, these skills are considered some of the building blocks of practice, with student midwives having to perfect them before being regarded as clinically competent. Until very recently, experience and skills in facilitating water births and physiological third stages of labour were not part of the curriculum.
- How many labour wards offer an established service of alternative therapies to support women in childbirth?

We will have to redefine 'normal practice' if we are to accept natural labour as 'normal'. Women often seek a natural, noninterventionalist birth and sadly, many come to the conclusion that they cannot achieve it. Only then do they look to alternatives. However, there is a rising trend in free birthing, with some women going to the extreme of birthing unattended in order to avoid intervention by professionals (Cooper and Clarke 2008).

It can be argued that for every free-birther, there is a woman who wants to have an elective caesarean section, to avoid labour completely. Birthing through an abdominal incision is fast becoming 'normal', and some argue that all women should have the choice of an elective section. Clearly, midwives must take some of the responsibility for the choices offered in terms of birthing place, pain relief and mode of delivery.

A number of organisations have recently attempted to define 'normal birth', including the Royal College of Midwives (RCM), the World Health Organization (WHO), the Royal College of Obstetricians and Gynaecologists (RCOG) and the Association for Improvements in the Maternity Services (AIMS). However, this complex debate is ongoing.

Who has the power to define normality?

Historically, obstetricians were the first to try and control childbirth, introducing the supine position for labour and founding midwifery schools as far back as the 17th century. Today, in the USA, obstetricians routinely attend at every birth.

However, this practice has been criticised by feminists such as Ina May Gaskin, who suggest that this paternalistic behaviour shows a lack of faith in women and their ability to give birth naturally. The profession has not been kind to alternative obstetricians, such as Wendy Savage (the women's rights campaigner), who hold unconventional views on childbirth, fertility and power and control in obstetrics.

When we consider the pioneers of childbirth, taking water birth as just one example, it is possible to come up with a long list of influential obstetricians — Frederick Leboyer, Igor Charkovsky and Michel Odent to name just three. Michel Odent went to enormous efforts to bring water birth into 'normal', everyday practice, making sure that he was present at every water birth in his area. It can be argued that obstetricians have the most influential role in defining normality.

This said, normality defines midwives and their practice, so is it not time that midwives reclaim 'normal birth' as their business? It is well documented that although invasive medical procedures are often used safely in labour, such procedures should only be performed where the benefit outweighs the harm (Dodwell 2010). Many practices that midwives undertake can increase the chances of women having normal births, through encouraging physiological processes. This chapter provides some of the tools to help you preserve normality during labour.

What is a normal birth?

The Maternity Care Working Party (MCWP) proposes a more precise definition of normal birth, to enable comparisons between different care delivery systems:

> *'A woman whose labour starts spontaneously, progresses spontaneously without drugs and who gives birth spontaneously'*
>
> *(RCM 2010)*

However, this definition still includes augmentation, artificial rupture of the membranes (when not a part of medical induction), postpartum haemorrhage, perineal repair, admission of the neonate to the SCBU or the NNU, the use of entonox or opioids and the use of electronic fetal monitoring to manage the third stage. The following are excluded:

- Induction of labour (with prostaglandins, oxytocics or artificial rupture of the membranes).

- Epidural and spinal anaesthesia.
- General anaesthesia.
- Forceps/ventouse extraction.
- Caesarean section.
- Episiotomy

You must keep abreast of any developments in defining normality, as some members of the MCWP would like to see the definition narrowed further, using terms such as 'physiological' and 'natural birth' (RCM 2010).

Some key points for helping labouring women are listed by Dodwell (2010):

- Build the woman's confidence in their ability to give birth.
- Make her feel valued.
- Actively listen to her — women need to be listened to.
- Help her to feel in control.
- Support women so they feel enriched by the experience and not traumatised.
- Provide an optimal birthing environment, which does not disturb the neuro-physical processes necessary for progress in labour.
- Enhance the woman's ability to cope with pain.

How can I do this to support women to have a normal labour and birth?

- Provide continuity of midwife-led care.
- Give the option of having the birth at home or in a birth centre.
- Offer birth preparation classes.
- Offer one-to-one care in labour.
- Encourage mobility and upright positions during labour.
- Offer access to immersion in water during labour, for pain relief.
- Consider the environment, particularly within the hospital (low lighting, quiet, safe).
- Being there counts. The woman and her partner need to be secure in the knowledge that you are there when needed.

Clarke *et al* (2007) suggest that all levels of staff should work together to promote normality, with an integrated pathway for natural birth. Following an audit, they found that more birth positions were used, more women experienced physiological third stage and more women went home directly from the birth centre. You should investigate whether or not your birthing unit has an integrated pathway for natural birth — if not, are they considering developing one?

What are signs of normal progress in labour?
Andi Simpson/Jacqui Williams

You must be in tune with the woman you are caring for. Recognising different behaviours will help you to encourage, support and comfort her throughout the labour. Labouring women are very vulnerable and need the support of birth partners. The traditional clinical criteria for progress in labour are:

- Length, strength and frequency of contractions.
- Effacement and dilatation of the cervix.
- Descent of the presenting part.
- Maternal and fetal condition.
- Congestion of the vulva.
- Dilation and gaping of anus.
- Perineal bulging.
- Rupture of membranes (that would normally remain intact until the second stage of labour)

However, what can you **observe** in the woman's behaviour which shows progress? The following are all possible:

- Restlessness.
- Changing facial expressions.
- Crying out, and making grunting noises.
- Vomiting.
- Irritability.
- Saying that she has an uncontrollable urge to push, or that she feels she is not in control.
- Withdrawal into herself.
- Sudden panic.

A crucial role of the midwife is to comfort the woman, and to reassure her throughout.

How can I improve my communication with women in labour?

Jethi Modhvadia

The presence of and physical contact with a midwife communicates many things to a labouring woman. It tells her that you are there with her, it provides reassurance and it can soothe her when she feels frightened. The majority of women need their partners or birth companions to remain close. Some will want physical contact in some shape or form, either constantly or occasionally, whereas others will want to be left alone. Compassion can be communicated as you wipe her brow, tie her hair up out of her face, help her to drink, provide ice chips, or physically assist her when she needs to change position. Your presence, your hands and your loving attitude are all very powerful support tools.

Most women make noises during labour. In the 1st stage, these can include inward and outward breathing, deeper sounds, releasing sounds (to match contractions) and towards the end of the 1st stage or transition, more rapid noises and at times higher-pitched squeals or screams (Devito 2001). During the 2nd stage, there may be moaning, groaning or grunting sounds from deep within the woman (Hall 2001), which many describe as 'primitive' and 'animalistic'. By making these sounds, women are able to release energy and tension from within their bodies and effectively move the fetus down the birth canal (Schott and Henley 1996). These noises are also a way for labouring women to indirectly communicate with the people around them. It is important that midwives are able to recognise all types of communication, including verbal, non-verbal, noises, body language and touch. As a midwife, you must create a private environment where the woman feels safe, so that she can behave instinctively without fear of being overheard or interrupted (Thompson 2003).

In terms of communication, you need to consider the following when caring for labouring women:

- The NMC Code (2008) states 'You must share with people, in a way they can understand, the information they want or need to know about their health.'
- Good, effective communication is an integral part of the midwife's role and central to all interactions with women and their families, and subsequently their experiences of midwifery care. Although verbal communication accounts for only a small percentage of overall communication, the words we use play a vital role in establishing the relationship and in power orientation of the birthing environment. (Devito 2001)

- Midwives need to provide continuous support to women with uncomplicated pregnancies during pregnancy in preparation for labour. Good communication between the midwife and the pregnant woman can help to reduce the risk for complications during childbirth. In communicating with the woman the midwife needs to pay special attention to the cultural values and personal preferences of the women in their care (Kitzinger 1997).
- A number of studies have shown communication difficulties to be the biggest source of complaint among childbearing women (McCourt 2006).
- Do not discourage her from making low-pitched sounds in labour. Pushing during the second stage is hard work and as the baby's head crowns, she may need to pant or even scream. Many women make these noises to enable them to work through the pain of labour.
- Never show irritation or frustration with the woman.
- If the woman is unable to understand the language you are using, try using non-verbal communication; consider learning a few key words in their language (Smith 2006).
- Work with the woman and not against her. Remember that you are her advocate — it is her pregnancy, her birth and she needs to decide what she wants. Your role is to provide her with the information to make informed decisions and to support her through her experience.
- Be mindful of the language you use — some words (e.g. 'just a ..' and 'little') can imply that procedures are routine and thus undermine a woman's feelings and concerns about what is happening to her (Thompson 2003).

To elaborate on this last point, a number of terms that are commonly used in midwifery can have a negative effect on women, such as 'failure to progress', 'patient', 'delivery suite', 'managing pain', 'pain relief' and 'refusing analgesia'. Using such terms in the questions and comments we make can cause women to feel disempowered, scared, angry and frustrated.

For example:

- Did you ring in?
- Are you in labour?
- Just hop on to the couch.
- I'm going to examine you.
- I'm going to help you feed your baby.
- You can't go home.
- This can go on for days.
- You're only in early labour.

Box 3.1 Pause for thought

Emma is having her second baby and is very anxious; she is 39 weeks pregnant and has had a normal pregnancy. Her cervix was 2cm dilated on an earlier admission to the hospital. Emma is now contracting 4 in 10 minutes and her waters have gone. Emma tried to ring the hospital a few times but the phone was engaged. She has arrived at the labour ward and is very anxious as she is arriving unannounced.

- What would you ask her on arrival?

- When would it be appropriate to discuss the importance of phoning before coming to the hospital? Is it important?

- Are you going to turn her away and ask her to ring and then come in?

We must ensure that the language we use with women in our care is appropriate and positive in nature. Mongan (2005) states that hypnobirthing techniques alter the language used into positive formulations:

- Babies are 'birthed' not 'delivered'.
- Membranes are 'released' not 'ruptured'.
- 'Birthing partners' or 'birthing companions'.
- Contractions are 'surges', denoted as steps towards the baby.
- 'Baby' not 'fetus'.

It is believed that words are associated with visualisations and emotions, which can dramatically affect outcomes.

What do I need to consider about food and fluids for women in labour?

Jethi Modhvadiu

Food is culturally important and has connections to both physical and psychological wellbeing. Historically, a number of substances have been used during labour for their supposed benefits, including alcohol, herbal potions, raw eggs, tea made from human hair and even gunpowder. In the western world, nutritional advice for labouring women changed following a 1946 publication by Mendelson and Parker, who argued that gastric emptying is slowed down during labour (Braoch and Newton 1998). This has since been disputed.

Newton and Champion's (1997) study of oral intake in labour at Nottingham City Hospital found that women who were given the choice of eating and drinking felt that they had more control over their labour. Further, they did not suffer from the discomfort of fasting, which is known to increase anxiety and stress in women. Stress is thought to have a number of undesirable effects on labour and on the baby's health, due to an excess of catecholamines, or stress hormones (adrenaline and noradrenalin) (Simkin 1986). In response to the physiological and psychological effects of childbirth, beta-endorphins are released, which regulate labour (Jowitt 1993) — under stress, they prolong it. They prevent oestrogen from 'wiring up' the uterus and they also reduce the secretion of oxytocin. They can reduce uterine efficiency, cause shunting of blood away from the uterus (reducing uteroplacental perfusion) and have effects on the fetal heart rate.

If no restrictions are enforced, women in all stages of labour seek some form of oral refreshment, including solid foods, although these needs decline as labour advances (Ludka and Roberts 1993). In a study in Ireland, births were an hour and a half quicker in women who ate during labour. These women required less pain relief and requested it much later compared with those who fasted. Less augmentation was required, and babies whose mothers had eaten while in labour were found to achieve better Apgar scores (a measure of newborn babies' health) (Gassidy 1999).

It could be argued that there is sufficient evidence to suggest that midwives should not discourage women from eating and drinking in low risk labours. However, there is a lack of evidence on whether fasting all labouring women affects morbidity or saves lives — women still die from Mendelson's syndrome, for instance, having been fasted and having received full antacid therapy during labour. There is scant information on factors which influence whether or not women eat during normal labour.

Tips for practice:

- Offer all low risk women the choice to eat and drink during labour.
- When contractions have decreased in their frequency, length or strength, consider foods such as honey water, dates, sugary fluids, biscuits, fruit juices, tea and toast.
- Drinking well during labour will prevent dehydration — it is the midwife and birth companions' job to remind the woman to drink. Give women water as and when they want it to avoid complicating a normal low risk labour.
- Remember that the body's priority is to meet its energy needs. If women fast during labour, energy will be generated from fat, protein and carbohydrate reserves (Champion and McCormick 2002).
- When women are not allowed to eat and drink in labour, ketone body levels can increase markedly and iatrogenic ketosis can occur (Anderson 1998).
- It is equally important that you not 'force feed' women. There is evidence to suggest that some ketones and free fatty acids can be advantageous to the progress of labour (Toohill *et al* 2003).
- Remember to both offer and try simple solutions first, before moving on to invasive and restricting options.
- Consider noninvasive ways of balancing ketone levels in low risk labours, for instance, with tea, toast, dates and biscuits.
- Consider light foods and fluids when women are tired during first and second stages of labour.

Scenarios to Consider:

1. Laura is 18 years old, primiparous, she is at term, has a low risk pregnancy, no medical history and is fit and well. Her cervix is 8cm dilated and her membranes are intact on admission. On transfer to the labour ward, her contractions decrease to 1 in 7 minutes.

What would you do?
What can cause a decrease in contractions?

2. Nichola is multiparous, she had a previous normal delivery, has a low-risk pregnancy and is at 37 weeks' gestation. On admission, her cervix was 4cm dilated and the membranes were intact. Four hours later, her cervix is 6cm dilated and the membranes remain intact. Her contractions cease and she is feeling very tired and losing the focus that she has had in labour until now.

What could be the reasons for this?
What would your action be?
Why might this have happened?

Much has been written on the importance of good nutrition during pregnancy and while breastfeeding, but most authors ignore the hours of labour and women's views on eating and drinking during labour. However, for the labouring woman, what she eats and drinks may be critical to her success giving birth. Most of us know what happens if expectant ladies don't eat — they get very 'crabby', 'shaky', nauseated and tend to lose their emotional control!

How should I monitor the fetal heart in low risk labours?
Jethi Modhvadia

Since its development in the 1960s, continuous electronic fetal monitoring (CEFM) has been a part of routine care during labour. By the 1980s, nearly half of all hospital labours were monitored continuously (Alfirevic *et al* 2006). Its proponents had hoped that, as a screening tool, CEFM technology would prevent fetal compromise or demise, decrease the incidence of cerebral palsy and reduce the number of lawsuits. However, to date it has failed to live up to these expectations (Deborah *et al* 2001).

We must consider the effect that fetal surveillance has had on women and birth companions, as CEFM reduces mobility and reduces contact with birth companions and with the midwife. Most babies go through labour with no problems and electronic fetal monitoring (EFM) is used to detect the few that have difficulty. Sometimes EFM is requested by the woman as it can provide reassurance, but it can also cause anxiety and distract focus during labour.

For low risk labours, intermittent auscultation is an option, although a thorough risk assessment should be performed for both the woman and fetus in order to appropriately identify suitable candidates (NICE 2007).

Successful intermittent monitoring can be achieved keeping in mind the following points:

- The skill and confidence of the midwife in auscultation technique, palpation of contractions, and recognition of fetal heart rate changes.
- Hospital policy and guidelines for technique and frequency of assessment.

- Appropriate action must be taken when findings are not within guidelines.
- One to one care is needed as the fetal heart must be monitored every 15 minutes in the first stage of labour and every 5 minutes in second stage of labour (NICE 2007).
- Variability can be difficult to determine.
- Never use a cardiotocograph (CTG) monitor to intermittently auscultate the fetal heart.
- Remember to document the labour both on the partogram and in the notes.

Structured intermittent auscultation of the fetal heart can be achieved with a handheld Doppler. Initially, abdominal palpation should be performed, then the Doppler can be placed over the fetal back (the maternal pulse should be checked to differentiate between the mother and baby). The fetal heart should then be auscultated for at least 60 seconds after contraction, to identify the fetal response to labour.

However, the primary instrument for intermittent auscultation is Pinnard's stethoscope. Although some women find the pressure necessary for good auscultation to be uncomfortable during labour, it has the advantage of only picking up the fetal heart sounds (and not the maternal pulse). To use the Pinnard, first palpate the abdomen to determine the fetal position and then place the bell of the Pinnard onto the abdomen. Press your ear on the flat end, to secure it, and then let go of the Pinnard and listen for muffled fetal heart sounds, similar to those heard when putting your ear onto an adult's chest (ARM 2011).

Things to consider during intermittent auscultation:

- How often should you be auscultating and for how long?
- Has the woman given her consent?
- Check the maternal pulse and palpate the uterine contractions.
- Have you determined the baseline fetal heart rate and its variability? Have you heard any accelerations or decelerations?
- Inform the woman of your findings, unless she has asked you not to.

Ultimately, if carried out correctly and competently, intermittent auscultation is cheap and noninvasive. Intermittent auscultation of the fetal heart does not interfere with the midwife and woman's relationship, trust and bonding, and healthy term fetuses need to be exposed to some stress in labour to prepare them for extra-uterine transition. EFM should be avoided for all low risk normal births and admissions (Hindley *et al* 2005). When deciding whether or not to use CEFM, you must evaluate the impact that it may have on the labouring woman and the restrictions on movement that it may cause.

What positions can promote normality in labour?

Andrea Simpson

Given freedom of movement, women choose a variety of positions during labour, which include standing, walking, rhythmic swaying, leaning forward, and on hands and knees. These positions are adopted in response to the pain and pressures of labour. It is well documented that labour progresses more efficiently when women respond to their body's cues and move accordingly to help the fetus find the 'best fit' through the pelvis. However, most hospital birthing rooms are set up such that the woman has to adapt to their attendant rather than the other way around. An increase in mobility and freedom of movement gives the woman back control over her labour and her space, which results in increased satisfaction with care.

Left to themselves, women in the first and second stages of normal labour tend to adopt positions that they find comfortable (Walsh 2007, Romano and Lothian 2008) — these do not necessarily involve a bed. However, most birthing/labour rooms have a bed in the centre of the room, lowered and with sheets arranged, so as to invite the woman to climb in (Cotton 2010). Once in bed, she may be reluctant to climb out again, perhaps feeling that she has to ask permission to change position. In fact, 91% of women give birth on a bed, with 56% in a recumbent position. Walsh (2007) goes so far as to say that beds should be removed from birthing rooms or pushed out of the way, recommending that furniture conducive to mobility and position changing be in the room instead, such as bean bags, birth balls, mats and birth stools

If you watch a woman during the course of her labour from the first contraction to birth and observe the positions she adopts, you will notice that she does not stay still. She starts out in a generally upright position — pacing, walking, leaning forward, dancing and swaying. As labour progresses, she gradually adopts a more forward-leaning posture, almost bowing, with her bow getting deeper and deeper until her legs start to give and bend during contractions. Gradually, she will move closer to the floor, either squatting or taking a position on her hands and knees, sometimes swaying. It is in this position that many women enter the second stage and the expulsive contractions begin. To be on a bed in a 'stranded beetle' position is not a part of this scene and is almost totally alien to the natural, inhibited birthing process. When the fetus passes over the rhombus of Michaelis, an 'all fours' position is ideal because as at this point, the pelvis becomes unstable. On all fours, the woman is able to stabilise herself. In contrast, in the stranded beetle position she will throw her arms up above her head and reach out to hold onto something, or grab the bed or chair to steady herself while the baby makes it passage past. NICE guidelines (2008) advise that women should be able to move freely and adopt whichever position suits them best during labour and birth, with support for more upright positions from the midwife or birth partner.

The pelvis is made of many bones and by adopting different positions, the woman can change its shape, allowing passage of the fetus during labour. It is possible for the woman to enlarge the front to back diameter and the transverse diameter, and the symphysis pubis and coccyx are able to flex backwards as much as 2cm. They can also flex forwards reducing the available space for the fetal head/presenting part.

There are many reasons why sitting on a coccyx is less than ideal. The obvious one is that it reduces the diameter of the pelvic outlet, which means there is less space for the fetus to move its head, to adopt the optimum position for birth. It can also prevent descent of the presenting part and deep engagement in the pelvis, which can cause a slower labour, increased perception of severe pain (resulting in epidural anaesthesia) and potentially augmentation of labour or instrumental delivery.

Why upright?

There is much evidence to show that upright positions are ideal for labour and birth and left to themselves, most women will adopt these positions.

Positive aspects of upright positions are:

- Shorter labour (by 90 minutes).
- Increased uterine contractility.
- Greater comfort for the labouring woman.
- Dancing and swaying can help a woman cope with the contractions.
- Decreased need for pharmacological pain relief (including epidural).
- Decreased need for augmentation of labour.
- Reduced occurrence of operative delivery.
- Less fetal distress and fetal heart rate abnormalities.
    (Adapted from Gupta et al 2004; Walsh 2007; Roman and Lothian 2008;
    Cotton 2010; Lawrence et al 2009)

There is no documented evidence of any harm from an upright position. In fact, there is plenty of evidence to show that movement and position changes can correct some complications in labour. For example:

- A premature urge to push.
- Some fetal heart abnormalities.
- Backache due to persistent posterior positioning (can be eased with the all fours position).
- Poor progress (can be improved with a more upright position).
- Malpositions such as occiput posterior or asynclitism (can be corrected by movement that changes the diameters of the pelvic outlet).

Changing position is the first line approach to correct complications when the mother and fetus are stable — for example, if the woman is supine, move her into the left lateral position (the supine position can cause aortocaval compression resulting in poor oxygenation of the fetus and reduced pH and Apgar score at birth).

What are the arguments for being upright and mobile?

- Gravity is increased, the second stage of labour is shorter, bearing down is easier (she can push against the pelvic floor), there are fewer episiotomies, fewer assisted births, less severe pain and reduced fetal heart abnormalities (better blood flow to the uterus, no aorto-caval compression).
- There is increased flexion and abduction of the hips and the coccyx is free to move backwards, increasing space at the pelvic outlet.
- The woman has increased control and ownership of the birth space.
- Upright positions include standing, kneeling, sitting up at >45 degrees, squatting (supported by the birth partner or by herself), sitting on a birth stool and forward leaning.
- Recumbent positions include supine, sitting at <45 degrees, lithotomy.
- Reasons against using beds: longer second stage, increased fetal heart abnormalities, increased interventions, reduced desire to bear down, reduced pelvic outlet diameter, more severe pain.

(Adapted from Gupta et al 2004)

What are the arguments against being in an upright position?

- Not all women want to be upright. When it comes to positioning, women must have a choice.
- As labour progresses, some women prefer to recline. They may find it difficult to be upright in the later parts of the first stage and in the second stage.

Tips for practice

Using a bed

- Turn the bed into a chair, so the woman is sat upright. Remove the base and if necessary, use the foot supports for something to push against.
- Put the back of the bed up and encourage the woman to lean over the back of the bed.
- Put the bed up high so the woman can use it to lean over.
- Lateral positions if the woman is unable to stand or be upright.

Without a bed

A variety of positions may be useful, including:

- Hands and knees on the floor.
- Squatting, supported by wall or bed (or partner).
- Standing with one foot up on a step and one on the floor — this opens the pelvis, which can be especially useful with an asynclitic birth (it makes more room for the fetus to adjust position). Asymmetrical kneeling also has the same effect.
- Using a birthing stool — this opens the pelvis, provides support and aids pushing in the second stage.
- Use a birthing ball as a moveable chair (the woman can hold onto the end of the bed) — this promotes widening of the pelvic diameters.
- Put a mat on the floor, then the woman can kneel over the ball. Encourage her to open her legs to widen the pelvic diameters (other mats on the floor can support her knees).

What do I need to consider when using water in normal labour?

Sue Nyombi

Since its first recorded use in the 1960s, water birth has become increasingly popular in many countries. Today, most maternity units in the UK have at least one birthing pool.

Women who have birthed their babies underwater often give positive reports, describing the experience as a very satisfying one. There is currently an expectation that maternity services should offer a water birth service and consequently, that midwives should be skilled in facilitating water births as part of their normal practice.

Over the years, the practice of water birth has been guided by a small amount of available evidence and by a multitude of media stories of drowning babies. This has led to professional anxiety and in some cases even fear — the risks of not maintaining the water temperature to within set boundaries, of managing maternal collapse in the water, of the cord snapping, of water embolism (to name but a few) can turn what should be a calmer birth experience into a critical event.

Fortunately, the research around water birth is ever increasing. As the knowledge base grows, the development of evidence-based guidelines becomes possible, which helps to ensure good practice. Due to the physiological effects of water immersion, water birth is now being explored as an option for high risk women, such as those with uterine scarring, hypertension and Group B Streptococcus (Benko 2009).

Physiological effects of water immersion on the mother:

* Increases relaxation.
* Decreases pain.
* Increase pelvic diameters.
* Increase buoyancy and mobility.
* Increase contractions.
* Increase oxytocin and endorphin production.
* Increases peripheral/muscle and skin temperature.
* Reduces blood pressure.
* Relaxes perineal tissue.
* Increases diuresis.
* Reduces noradrenaline and adrenaline.

Physiological effects of water immersion on the fetus:

* Reduced gravitational pull at birth.
* Reduced exposure to pharmacological analgesia.
* There is some suggestion that water provides a gentler transition from intra- to extra-uterine life and a slower adjustment of circulation at birth.
* The baby appears quieter and calmer at birth.

Water birth risks — truth or myth?

'The baby might breathe underwater.'

This has been associated both with the baby being externally stimulated when immersed underwater, and with fetal distress.

Environmental and physiological reasons have been cited to explain why babies do not breathe underwater. Garland (2000) explores how the immersed environment mimics that of the uterus and consequently delays respiration until the baby is exposed to air — water birth takes place in a reduced gravityenvironment, the baby receives no stimulation (a non-touch technique is used), the umbilical cord is not clamped and cut before exposure to air, and the water temperature is maintained close to body temperature.

Harper (2000) goes further, explaining that the baby has in-built inhibitory factors that prevent underwater breathing. These include the suppression of fetal breathing before labour begins and also the hypoxic response to birth — hypoxia causes apnea and swallowing, not breathing or gasping. Having said this, if the fetus were experiencing a severe and prolonged lack of oxygen, then theoretically it may gasp as soon as it was born, possibly inhaling water into the lungs. Hence, the woman should exit the pool if fetal distress is suspected.

The 'dive reflex' protects the lungs as when a solution hits the back of the throat, passing the larynx, the glottis automatically closes and the solution is then swallowed, not inhaled. Furthermore, as water is hypotonic and the fetal lung fluids are hypertonic, even if water were to travel in past the larynx, then it could not pass into the lungs — hypertonic solutions are denser and prevent hypotonic solutions from merging or coming into their presence.

'Strict water temperature guidelines are necessary'

Many guidelines include rigorous control of water temperature, due to a fear of causing fetal hypoxia if the water is too hot, or of stimulating underwater breathing (freshwater drowning) if it is too cold.

The NICE Guidelines (2007) state that the temperature of both the woman and the water should be monitored hourly, to ensure that the woman is comfortable and not becoming pyrexial.

The water temperature should not be allowed to rise above 37.5°C as this will cause the mother's temperature to rise and, in turn, the fetus's. Beyond 38°C, the fetus's oxygen requirements can increase and if not met, the fetus will become hypoxic and may be compromised.

In 2002 Barbara Harper challenged the British obsession with temperature regulation stating that it should be maintained at what is comfortable for the woman. This was following the birth of a baby who was born into the Mediterranean Sea with an estimated temperature of 24 degrees centigrade, with no apparent ill effects.

A study by Geissbuehler *et al* (2002) gave women free choice on water temperature without any upper or lower limits. The results are intriguing — compared with those born on land, water birth babies had lower morbidity, improved cord pH and Apgar scores, less respiratory distress and fewer NICU admissions. The water temperatures ranged from 23–38.8°C and the women spent between 28 and 364 minutes in the pool.

For a naked human, the neutral comfort zone (the point at which neither sweat glands nor heat formation mechanisms are activated) is usually 28°C in air, or 35–36°C in water. However, the exact temperature depends on how much adipose tissue a person has — in people with thick layers of fat, it has been found to be as low as 31 degrees. With this in mind, Geissbuehler *et al* (2002) argue that strict water temperature guidelines could dangerously disrupt individuals' physiological temperature control circuits. They suggest that we focus our attention on making the woman feel comfortable, and ensuring that she has control over her environment.

'There is an increased chance of the cord snapping during a water birth?'

There have been reports of increased cord snapping at water births but as yet there is no explanation as to why. Some strategies have been suggested to reduce the risk at water birth, such as ensuring the water is not unnecessarily deep during the second stage, bringing the baby gently to the surface, having cord clamps to hand and delivering the baby completely underwater (before lifting to the surface). You should remember that cord snapping is a rare occurrence. However, it happens in both land and water births and visibility can be difficult in water. The immediate assessment of the cord at birth should be a part of routine care with water births.

Box 3.2 Practice point

Take the opportunity to work with midwives who are experienced in water birth and attend a practical workshop. This will give you the skills and confidence to offer this option to women in your care.

In summary

- The physiological effects of water birth, both maternal and fetal, make it a popular choice.
- There are both environmental and physiological reasons for why babies do not breathe underwater.
- Guidelines on water temperature may be detrimental to the physiological temperature control circuit — we should adjust the water temperature to the woman's comfort.
- Cord snapping, although rare, is slightly increased at water births. Therefore, close observation of the cord at birth is recommended.

Is music useful in for women in labour?

Jacqui Williams

We often ask labouring women if they would like to listen to music, and music is often played in theatre. Its effects on pain and anxiety during labour have been examined by a recent Taiwanese study (Liu *et al* 2010), which found it to be an acceptable, non-medical coping strategy that did reduce pain and anxiety in the early phases of labour. However, this study failed to state how music was chosen, which may be a crucial consideration. Nevertheless, this study reminds us that we must build on the little work that has been done in this area.

You should think about using music in labour and encourage women to bring in their own choices of music with them. This should include some that can be listened to with headphones, so they can listen without being distracted by other noises in the environment.

References

Alfirevic Z, Devane D, Gyte GML (2006) Continuous cardiotocography (CTG) as a form of electronic fetal monitoring (EFM) for fetal assessment during labour. *Cochrane Database Syst Rev.* **19(3):** CD006066

Anderson T (1998) Is Ketosis in Labour Pathological? *Pract Midwife.* **1(9):** 22-6.

Association of Radical Midwives (ARM) (2011) www.midwifery.org.uk (accessed 3/4/11)

Benko A (2009) Waterbirth: Is it a real choice? *Midwifery Matters* **22:** 9-12

Braoch J, Newton N (1988) Food and Beverages in Labour. Part 1: Cross Cultural and Historical Practices. *Birth.* **15(2):** 81–5.

Clarke P, Bowcock M, Gales P (2007) Development of an Integrated Care Pathway for Natural Birth. *Br J Midwifery.* **15(1):** 12-15

Champion P, McCormick C (2002) *Eating and drinking in labour.* Butterworth-Heinemann, Oxford

Cooper T, Clarke P (2008) Freebirthing: home alone: a concerning trend. *Midwives.* **11(3):** 34-5

Cotton J (2010) Considering the evidence for upright positions in labour. MIDIRS *Midwifery Digest* **20(4):** 459- 463

Department of Health (2004) National Health Service Maternity Statistics 2002–2003. www.publications.doh.gov.uk/public/sb0410.pdf (accessed 3/4/11)

Devito J A (2001) *Essentials of Human Communication. 4th edn.* Addison-Wesley, Harlow.

Dodwell M (2010) *Normal birth as a measure of quality of care.* National Childbirth Trust (NCT), London

Downe S (2008) *Normal Childbirth: Evidence and Debate. 2nd edn.* Churchill Livingstone, Edinburgh.

Garland D (2000) *Waterbirth – an attitude to care.* Books for Midwives, Oxford.

Gassidy P (1999) Management of The First Stage of Labour. In: Bennett V R, Brown L K (eds) *Myles textbook for midwives. 13th edn.* Churchill Livingstone, Edinburgh.

Geissbuehler V; Stein S; Eberhard J (2004).Waterbirths compared with landbirths: an observational study of nine years. *J Perinat Med.* **32(4):** 308-314

Gupta J K, Hofmeyr G J (2004). Position for women during second stage of labour. *Cochrane Database Syst Rev.* **(1):** CD0020006

Hall J (2001) *Midwifery mind and spirit: emerging issues of care.* Books for midwives, Oxford.

Harper B (2000) Waterbirth Basics – From Newborn Breathing to Hospital Protocols. *Midwifery Today.* **54:** 9-15, 68.

Harper B (2002) Taking the plunge: re-evaluating waterbirth temperature guidelines. MIDIRS *Midwifery Digest.* **12(4):** 506-8

Hindley C, Wren Hinsliff S, Thompson A M (2005) English midwives views and experiences of intrapartum fetal heart rate monitoring in women at low obstetric risk: conflicts and compromises. *J Midwifery Women's Health.* **51(5):** 354–360.

Jowitt M (1993) Beta-endorphin and stress in pregnancy and labour. *Midwifery Matters.* **56:** 3–4.

Lawrence A, Lewis L, Hofmeyr GJ, Dowswell T, Styles C (2009). Maternal positions and mobility during first stage labour. *Cochrane Database Syst Rev.* **2:** CD003934

Ludka L M, Roberts C (1993) Eating and Drinking in Labour: A literature review. *J Nurse Midwifery.* **38(4):** 199–207.

Lui Y H, Chang M Y, Chen C H (2010) Effects of music therapy on labour pain and anxiety in Taiwanese first-time mothers. *J Clin Nursing.* **19(7-8):** 1065-1072

Kitzinger S (1997) Authoritative touch in childbirth – A cross cultural approach. In: Davis-Floyd R E, Sargent C F (eds) *Childbirth and authoritative knowledge: cross cultural perspective.* University of California Press, Berkeley

Midwifery 2020 Programme (2010) Midwifery 2020 Delivery Expectations September www.midwifery2020.org (accessed 5/1/11)

McCourt C (2006) Supporting choice and control? Communication and interaction between midwives and the women at the antenatal booking visit. *Soc Sci Med.* **62(6):** 1307–1318.

Mongan F (2005) *Hypnobirthing: the Mongan Method. 3rd edn.* Health Communications.

Munro J (2008) *Positions for labour and birth – a midwifery practice guideline.* Royal College of Midwives, London

National Collaborating Centre for Women's and Children's Health (2008) *Intrapartum Care: care of healthy women and babies during childbirth.* RCOG Press, London

NCT/RCM/RCOG (2007) Making normal birth a reality: Consensus statement from the Maternity Care Working Party our shared views about the need to recognise, facilitate and audit normal birth. www.rcm.org.uk/college-archive/resources/campaign-for-normal-birth/

National Institute for Health and Clinical Excellence (NICE) (2007) *Clinical guidance 55: intrapartum care.* London National Institute for Health and Clinical Excellence.

Newton and Champion (1997) Oral Intake in Labour: Nottingham's Policy Formulated and Audited. *Br J Midwifery.* **5(7):** 418-422

Nursing and Midwifery Council (2008) *The code: Standards of conduct, performance and ethics for nurses and midwives.* NMC, London

Romano AM, Lothian JA (2008) Promoting, protecting and supporting normal birth: a look at the evidence. *J Obstet Gynecol and Neonatal Nurs* **37(1):** 94-105

Royal College of Midwives (RCM) (2010) *Making normal birth a reality Consensus statement from Maternity Care Working Party.* RCM, London. www.rcm.org.uk (accessed 3/4/11)

Schott J, Henley A (1996) *Culture and religion and childbearing in a multiracial society: a handbook for health professionals.* Butterworth-Heinemann, Oxford.

Simpkin P (1986) Stress, Pain and catecholamines in labour, Part 2. Stress events associated with childbearing events: a pilot survey of new mothers. *Birth.* **13(4):** 234–240.

Smith S (2006) Cross cultural information leaflets. *Nurs Stand.* **21(4):** 39-41

Thompson N (2003) *Communication and Language: a handbook of theory and practice.* Palgrave Macmillan, London.

Toohill J, Soong B, Flenady V (2003) Interventions for Ketosis During Labour. *Cochrane Database Syst Rev.* CD004230.

Walker DS, Shunkwiler S, Supanich J, Williamsen J, Yensch A (2001) Labour and delivery nurses attitudes toward intermittent fetal monitoring. *J Midwifery Women's Health.* **46(6):** 374–380.

Walsh D (2007) *Mobility and Posture in Labour in Evidence-based care for normal labour and birth: A guide for midwives.* Routledge, London.

Chapter 4

Developing and enhancing midwifery skills

- **What is interprofessional working in midwifery practice?**
- **What are the principles of interpreting cardiotocograph (CTG) traces?**
- **What is fetal heart classification?**
- **What care should I give to a woman following a lower segment caesarean section (LSCS)?**
- **What do I need to consider when caring for a woman with an epidural?**
- **What are the principles of safe practice for giving medication?**
- **What are the principles of drug administration in midwifery?**
- **How can I ensure that my drug calculations are correct?**
- **How can I calculate the mean arterial pressure (MAP)?**
- **How can I calculate the body mass index (BMI)?**
- **How can I avoid drug errors?**

What is interprofessional working in midwifery practice?
Jacqui Williams

> *'Midwives will be the lead professional for all healthy women with straightforward pregnancies. For women with complex pregnancies they will work as the key coordinator of care with the multidisciplinary team, liaising closely with obstetricians, general practitioners, health visitors/public health practitioners and maternity support workers/maternity care assistants.'*
>
> *Midwifery 2020 Programme (2010)*

A modern NHS needs professionals 'to work collaboratively and form partnerships to ensure seamless delivery of care' (Cullen 2003). In accordance with Nursing and Midwifery Council (NMC) standards, practising midwives are responsible for providing women and babies with midwifery care during the antenatal, intranatal and postnatal periods and 'cannot arrange for anyone to act as a substitute other than another registered midwife or registered medical practitioner' (NMC 2006). However, a modern NHS needs professionals 'to work collaboratively and form partnerships to ensure seamless delivery of care' (Cullen 2003).

Multiprofessional development and training is encouraged, with regular skills training and drills to maintain competence. The World Health Organisation (WHO) has long proposed that complex problems within healthcare can be better solved when health professionals have learnt together (WHO 1984) and the Royal College of Obstetricians and Gynaecologists (RCOG) (2007) further acknowledges the importance of team-working and effective communication channels.

Care should be a team effort, yet in the classroom and the workplace, the focus tends to be on individual professionals' contributions. It has long been recognised that interprofessional teams offer greater staff efficiency and more effective service provision (McGrath 1991). Leathard (2003) argues that the recognition of commonality between professions is central to effective collaboration in care delivery.

To work interprofessionally, practitioners must have a clear understanding of different professional roles, both their own and those of other professionals (Bainbridge *et al* 2010). After qualifying, you must continue to develop your competencies to ensure you are up to date with current evidence-based midwifery.

'A High Quality Workforce: NHS Next Stage Review' (Department of Health [DoH] 2008) recognises that the provision of care is a team activity. It is this acknowledgement that will allow us to move interprofessional working forward.

A flexible workforce

The need for a 'flexible' workforce was highlighted in both 'The new NHS, modern and dependable' (DoH 1998) and 'The NHS Plan' (DoH 2000) and is a goal that we, as professionals, have striven towards. However, those from different backgrounds (clinical, educational or governmental) may have been pursuing different criteria. If we are to achieve a flexible workforce, we must first define what is meant by 'flexible'.

The Concise Oxford Dictionary (2001) defines 'flexible' as 'readily adaptable', which is likely how professionals with a clinical or governmental focus have judged flexibility. Most NHS workforce planning documentation discusses the need for flexibility in working times and service provision, but there is no specific guidance as to how this might be achieved — perhaps understandably, as every healthcare provider can argue that their circumstances are unique to their clientele.

What is clear is that to be flexible a midwife must understand the principles of teamwork and the importance of collaboration.

What are the principles of interpreting cardiotocograph (CTG) traces?

Jacqui Williams

During active labour the fetal heart rate should be recorded every 15 minutes, for a full minute following a contraction. It is important to document the method of auscultation you are using.

The National Health Service Litigation Authority (NHSLA) requires that fetal heart training be done every 6 months (NHLSA 2011) and as a qualified midwife you are accountable to provide evidence that you have achieved this. Each year, your Trust will address this at an obstetric training day that you will attend. You will also undertake less formal training in the interim, which may include personal reading and review, reflection on a case study for your portfolio, follow up of a community referral, discussion of a CTG trace at an intrapartum meeting, following a ward round, attendance at a study day, or completion of the 'CTG Tutor' on www.perinatal.nhs.uk

What is fetal heart classification?

Jacqui Williams

If you are using continuous fetal monitoring, you will need to categorise and record whether the trace is 'normal', 'suspicious' or 'pathological'. The table below (Table 4.1) can help you determine which category the trace fits into and the plan of action required.

Table 4.1 Classification of fetal heart rate traces

Feature	Baseline (bpm)	Variability (bpm)	Decelerations	Accelerations
Reassuring	110–160	≥5	None	Present
Non-reassuring	100-109 161-180	≤5 for 40–90 mins	Typical variable decelerations with over 50% of contractions, occurring for over 90 minutes.	The absence of accelerations with otherwise normal trace is of uncertain significance.
Abnormal	<100 >180 Sinusoidal pattern ≥10 mins	<5 for 90 mins	Either atypical variable decelerations with over 50% of contractions or late decelerations, both for over 30 mins Single prolonged deceleration for more than 3 mins	

Source: NICE (2007) Classification of foetal heart rate/definition of normal, suspicious and pathological foetal heart traces

Table 4.2 Key terms for reviewing a cardiotocograph (CTG) trace of a fetal heart

Make sure you can write a definition for each

Baseline fetal heart
Normal baseline
Moderate bradycardia
Abnormal bradycardia
Abnormal tachycardia
Baseline variability
Normal baseline variability
Non-reassuring baseline variability
Accelerations
Decelerations
Early decelerations
Late decelerations
Variable decelerations
Atypical variable decelerations
Prolonged decelerations
Sinusoidal pattern

Remember that the most important thing to document in the notes is your plan. A useful template is the following:

- Date/time
- Baseline
- Variability
- Decelerations
- Accelerations
- Plan
- Sign and print name and designation

What care should I give to a woman following a lower segment caesarean section (LSCS)?

Jacqui Williams

Adapted from NICE Clinical Guideline 13: Caesarean Section (2004)

In the UK, the rate of lower segment caesarean section (LSCS) has risen — in 1980, it was 9% and by 2008–9 it had reached 24.6%. (Bragg *et al* 2010). Midwives regularly have to care for women following both elective and emergency caesarean sections. A caesarean should still be a positive experience for the woman and her partner and they should be offered a range of choices postnatally.

The handover from the delivery suite to the postnatal ward is vital. This must establish not only the woman's physical requirements, such as thromboprophylaxis or removal of an epidural catheter (if still *in situ*) but also her psycho-social needs. You should find out what occurred during labour, and what the woman's aspirations for labour and delivery had been.

Physical care

On admission to the postnatal ward, there should be an initial review during which the woman's vital signs should be recorded (temperature, pulse, respiration rate and blood pressure). Once stable, hourly observations need to be taken, including assessment of the following:

- Intravenous fluid regime and regular review of the cannula site. The intravenous catheter will usually be removed once oral fluids are tolerated but not earlier than 12 hours following surgery.
- Check the wound for any leakage through the dressing, initially and at regular intervals during the first 12 hours. The dressing can be removed the day after the operation and you should continue to observe for any signs of infection (pain, redness, discharge, separation, dehiscence). The woman needs to be advised on cleanliness and comfort, e.g. patting dry with a clean cloth (such as a separate towel or tissue) following a shower and ensuring that underwear does not rub on the suture line. You should encourage her to take regular analgesia to maintain adequate pain relief. If necessary, sutures or staples will be removed five days after surgery.
- Assess lochia for the amount present.

- Check that her Foley catheter is on straight drainage. Once the woman is mobile, this can be removed.
- Ensure that her fluid balance is monitored, particularly urinary output until discharge, or for at least 72 hours post caesarean section. Following catheter removal, measure the initial urine output to ensure that this is adequate.
- When aditted to the ward, how is the woman in herself? Is she sleepy? In any pain? Ensure that adequate pain relief is prescribed and offered at four-hourly intervals and assess how she is coping and recovering.
  - In theatre, diclonefac 100mg per rectum is usually given (provided there are no contraindications, such as aspirin allergy)
  - Thereafter, paracetamol 1g is given orally four times daily as well as diclofenac 50mg orally three times a day, or 100mg twice a day. The first oral dose is to be given 12 hours after the initial dose in theatre.
  - Other drugs that may be given as required include dihydrocodeine 30mg, orally, four-hourly or tramadol 50–100mg, orally, four-hourly.
  - The woman should also be given analgesia to take home, such as co-codamol 2 tablets orally, as required, or diclofenac 50mg orally three times a day, as necessary.
- Risk assess the woman's pressure areas using the Waterlow scoring system.
- The woman needs to be gently encouraged to mobilise no later than 24 hours following the LSCS, but not within 12 hours of the last epidural top-up. The day after surgery, a physiotherapy review can assist with mobilisation and breathing exercises.
- An obstetric review will be required 24–48 hours after the LSCS.
- All care must carefully documented, as contemporaneously as is possible (NMC 2004)

(adapted from NICE guidelines 2004)

Other important aspects of care

Although LSCS is a common occurrence, you mustn't forget that this is a major operation and the woman will need time to recover. She will also be adapting to parenthood and the demands of a newborn baby. The Caesarean Organisation (www.caesarean.org.uk) reports that a significant number of women who have undergone a first LSCS report that their baby does not feel like theirs. Although these women know that the baby really is theirs, they may not be in control of what they feel. Consider the following example:

'Never mind dear, have this one. It's better that one you had anyway.'
'It feels like I picked him up in Sainsbury's somehow – but I can't take him back.'
(Lowdon 1995)

Lowdon (1995) stresses that this traumatic reaction and its associated feelings of failure and grief need to be understood. She also argues that this reaction needs to be respected — midwives must empathise with women and not trivialise how they are feeling. The midwife can play an important role in supporting women who have negative feelings following a LSCS. Lowdon (1995b) also provides some useful questions to ask women in the days and months following a caesarean section. For example:

• Were you awake during the caesarean?
• Was it planned or was it an emergency?
• Did you have a general anaesthetic?

This information will already be available for the women in your care but these questions can help to shift the focus away from the 'whys' and 'wherefores', which can undermine a woman's confidence as she becomes preoccupied with 'where it went wrong'. Of course, many women will not feel disappointed that they did not give birth vaginally. However, you must ensure that women are not made to feel that they have 'failed' by not giving birth vaginally, by making insensitive comments or asking inappropriate questions.

What can you do to enhance her care?

During her time on the ward, ensure that the woman is observed regularly and that she always has a call button to hand — rooming in will still be encouraged and she may even be in a side room. She should feel that she has enough support and care, as women can feel very frightened if left alone for any length of time. She will need support with her baby but you should still encourage her to be involved in the care of her newborn.

It can be particularly important to women who have had a LSCS and wish to breastfeed that they succeed. For first-time mothers, breastfeeding can be more of a challenge than expected, and a LSCS can present more challenges. Newburn and Doods (2010) cite Raphael's work (1973), which describes 'matraescence' (the process of becoming a mother) as a major life crisis — this seems relevant when considering LSCS recovery. Following LSCS, women need support to breastfeed and to adjust to motherhood. You must give these women time and respond to their individual needs in an unhurried manner.

What do I need to consider when caring for a woman with an epidural?

Jacqui Williams

Epidural analgesia is an increasingly popular choice for pain relief in labour, particularly among primigravidae. While it has some very positive attributes (when used for LSCS, it is possible to avoid the risks of general anaesthesia), you must clearly communicate both its positive and negative effects so that women can make informed choices when deciding whether or not to request it.

Some authors question the use of epidural in normal labour (Lavender and Kingdon 2006; World Health Organisation 1996) — a debate that centres around society's perception of pain as abnormal, viewing it in the same way as pain that is associated with illness (Carne 2009).

While an epidural can offer good pain relief, will the woman be satisfied with her birth experience? It has previously been reported that women with an epidural *in situ* do not report birth as a positive experience (Morgan *et al* 1982).

Its effects on breastfeeding are still unclear. Some authors suggest that good breastfeeding support is crucial (Reynolds 2010; Devroe *et al* 2009) and others argue that there is evidence to show that epidural hinders breastfeeding (Rioidan, 1999). Indeed, Beilin *et al* (2005) found that women who received higher doses of fentanyl were more likely to have stopped breastfeeding at six weeks' postpartum.

It is acknowledged that the pain of childbirth can be very painful, but is epidural the answer? Using an epidural for pain relief in labour can lead to a 'cascade of interventions'.

Care considerations include:

- Level of pain.
- Level of block.
- Giving top ups in a timely manner (if epidural is not continuous).
- Maintenance of intravenous fluids.
- Maintenance of the woman's comfort (her movement is restricted), particularly in relation to warmth.
- Bladder care.

- Measuring vital signs, particularly blood pressure, pulse and temperature (body temperature can rise as a result of epidural, often during the first hour). You must ensure that the anaesthetist is informed of any changes.
- Continuous fetal monitoring and uterine activity — on the graph, you should indicate details that relate to the epidural, e.g. siting, top ups.
- Normal care should continue, recognising progress and any deviations from normal.
- Involve the woman in all aspects of her care.
- She needs clear instructions and advice — particularly during the second stage and delivery if she does not have full movement or feeling.
- Pressure area care — a woman's position should be changed every 1–2 hours.
- Although the evidence is mixed, there are possible effects on the newborn.
- Ensure that records are kept in line with NMC Rule 6 (NMC 2004).
- The epidural must be removed correctly postnatally.

Midwives who are trained and supervised can give top ups while adhering to local policy.

What are the principles of safe practice for giving medication?

Annie Law/Jacqui Williams

The NMC's Standards for Medicine Management (2008) outlines the minimum standards of practice for giving medication and should be used in conjunction with your local policies and procedures.

Midwives should incorporate the five 'rights' of drug administration into their practice:

- Use the right drug.
- Give to the right woman.
- Give the right dose.
- Give by the right route.
- Give at the right time.

(Nursing Times 1994)

The following (Table 4.3) is a step by step guide to the stages that you should follow in the checking and administration of drugs:

Table 4.3 Drug administration flow chart

Action	Rationale
Before administration, read prescription chart carefully. Ensure that you know what the drug is for, the usual dose, side-effects, contraindications and any special instructions or precautions	To check that the prescription is written clearly and accurately (in indelible ink). It is part of the nurse's role is to act as the last line of defence against errors. The doctor may have overlooked potential interactions and may have made a mistake in the dose or route (*Nursing Times* 1994b; NMC 2008)
If prescription chart is unclear in any way, return to prescriber for clarification	To reduce the risk of error (Dimond, 2004; Nursing Times, 1994b)
Check that the patient's details are clearly written on the chart. If there are patients with the same or similar name, a warning label should be attached to the chart	To provide sufficient information to check that medicines are given to the correct patient
If more than one chart, ensure that charts are clearly marked 1 of 2, or 2 of 2, as appropriate – merge all onto one chart at earliest opportunity	Ensures that everyone is aware of the existence of more than one chart to reduce the risk of missed doses
Check that the patient's weight is clearly written if any medicine is prescribed where the dose is related to weight	
Check each prescription for: • Name of drug • Route of administration • Dose • Start date • Signature of doctor • Any special instructions (e.g. with food) • Time of last administration • Time due for administration (NMC 2008)	To ensure that the correct drug is given by the correct route in the right dose at the right time. Some drugs, e.g. antibiotics, are only given for a short course; as the nurse administering the drugs you should request a review of the need for a drug if it has been given for longer *table continued overleaf.*

Table 4.3 [continued]

Check for any coexisting therapy, particularly in the 'as required' section	To ensure the same drug or constituent of a drug has not been prescribed in more than one section – risk of overdose (NMC 2008)
Check drug against prescription: • Name of drug • Dose of tablet/capsule/syrup, etc • Calculation (if any) • Expiry date (NMC 2008)	To ensure that correct dose and drug is given
Check patient's identity against prescription chart and name bracelet. Always ask the patient to state their name, address and date of birth; do not ask 'Are you Mr ....', as a confused, hard-of-hearing, or anxious patient may answer yes to this question when it is not his/her identity	To ensure that correct patient receives the correct drug (*Nursing Times* 1994b; NMC 2008)
Obtain patient's consent and administer the drug	Patient's consent is required for all treatments (NMC 2008)
Record that the drug has been administered. Where supervising a student in the administration of medicines, you should clearly countersign the signature of the student (NMC, 2008)	To indicate that the drug has been given and to prevent the dose being given again
Record if the drug has not been given for any reason and inform the prescriber	It may be necessary to alter the route of administration or review the need for the drug (NMC, 2008)
Instruction by telephone to administer a previously unprescribed substance is not acceptable (NMC, 2008)	Risk of unclear instructions or misunderstanding. If absolutely necessary, repeat instructions back to prescriber and ensure that you have a second witness; both of you should record the instructions

What are the principles of drug administration in midwifery?

Jacqui Williams

Under the Medicines Act 1968, midwives are exempt from certain restrictions on the sale or supply and administration of medicines. This unique role of the midwife follows advice given in the Crown Report (1998) and the Health Service Circular 'Patient Group Directions' (DoH 2000).

Midwives may supply or administer medicines to women in their care in the following circumstances:

- When it is a midwifery exempt drug.
- Under a Patient Group Direction.
- Against a prescription signed by an authorised prescriber.

However, NHS Trusts demand that training and an assessment be undertaken before midwives can administer medication.

I. Midwifery exempt drugs:

1.1 Under The Medicines Act 1968, medicines are divided into three categories:

- General Sales List (GSL)
- Pharmacy only (P)
- Prescription Only Medicines (POM)

1.2 Midwives may legally supply or administer all GSL and P medicines and certain POMs in the course of their professional practice.

1.3 Within each Trust, there is a list of midwifery exempt drugs that midwives may supply or administer to women in their care once training has been given and authorisation to administer medicines under a PGD has been granted.

1.4 Indications and dosages must be in line with recommendations in the current edition of the British National Formulary (BNF), or with trust guidelines.

Patient group directions

> 'Patients group directions are 'written instructions for the supply and/or administration of a licensed medicine (or medicines) in an identified clinical situation signed by a doctor or dentist and a pharmacist'. They apply to groups of patients who may not be individually identified before presenting for treatment.'
>
> *(National Prescribing Centre 2009)*

A PGD is a specific written instruction for the supply or administration of a named medicine (or medicines) in an identified clinical situation. It is drawn up locally by doctors, pharmacists and other appropriate professionals and then approved by the Trust. After ruling out any contraindications, the medicines included in a PGD policy may be dispensed as a once only dose to 'adult' patients (over 16 years), unless otherwise stated in the individual drug profile.

The NMC's Standards for Medicines Management (2008) states that a PGD can only be used by a midwife who has been assessed as competent to do so. Each PGD identifies a list of competent midwives, so delegation is not possible. Therefore, student midwives cannot supply or administer medicines under a PGD. Nonetheless, they are expected to understand the principles and be involved in the process (NMC 2009).

Some Trusts are implementing triennial drug assessments, e.g. practical observation of drug administration and multiple choice questions, testing knowledge of relevant policies, regulations and drug calculations.

How do I know what I can administer?

Legislation is very clear about how a PGD should be produced. It should include:
- The clinical condition covered by the direction.
- A description of those patients excluded from treatment under the direction.
- A description of the circumstances under which further advice should be sought from a doctor and referral arrangements be made.
- Appropriate dosage and maximum total dose, quantity, pharmaceutical form, strength, route, frequency of administration and the minimum or maximum period over which the medicine should be administered.
- Relevant warnings, including potential adverse reactions.
- Details of any follow-up action and the circumstances.
- A statement of the records to be kept for audit purposes.

(National Prescribing Centre 2009)

Implications for midwifery:

- Always check the prescription carefully against the drug to be given.
- Check the woman's identity against the prescription chart, even if it is some-one you know well.
- Be assertive to prevent interruptions, until you have administered the drug.
- Always follow local policies and procedures — they are there to protect the woman form harm and yourself form errors
- If you do make an error, report it immediately to minimise harm to the woman.

Exemptions are very different from prescribing. A midwife can only prescribe if she has completed a NMC-approved prescriber course and this is recorded on the NMC register. In June 2010 there were changes to the Midwives exemption list, so it is important that you keep up to date with current legislation (Homeyard and Forrester 2011).

How can I ensure my drug calculations are correct?
Annie Law/Jacqui Williams

'Some drug administrations require complex calculations to ensure that the correct volume or quantity of medication is administrated. In these situations, it is good practice for a second practitioner (a registered professional) to check the calculation independently, in order to minimise the risk of error. The use of calculators ....should not act as a substitute for arithmetical knowledge and skill.'
(NMC 2007)

When starting your first post, your Trust will require that you complete a training package. You must acquire an in depth knowledge of the medication

---

Table 4.4 A reminder about measurements

Mega- a million of a unit ($\times 10^6$)
Kilo- a thousand of a unit ($\times 10^3$)
Milli- a thousandth of a unit ($\times 10^{-3}$)
Micro- a millionth of a unit ($\times 10^{-6}$)
Nano a billionth of a unit ($\times 10^{-9}$)

Table 4.5 Some common conversions

I kilogram (kg)	=	1000 grams (g)
I gram (g)	=	1000 milligrams (mg)
I milligram (mg)	=	1000 micrograms (µg)
I litre (L or l)	=	1000 millilitres (ml)
I mole (mol)	=	1000 millimoles (mmol)
I millimole (mmol)	=	1000 micromoles (mcmol)

regularly used in your own area of practice and you must be familiar with your local Trust's medicines policy.

Liquid volumes are often expressed in millilitres (ml) and medication doses are often expressed in milligrams (mg). These are two of the most common units that your calculations will involve.

Can you convert the following?

- **324g**   (g?)   (mg?)
- **23mg**   (g?)   (µg?)
- **7400µg**   (mg?)   (g?)

Doses should always be in the same units.

When ordering medication, you should do your best to order tablets of the correct strength and use as few as possible. Try to use whole tablets, only breaking a tablet in half if it is scored down the middle, to ensure an accurate dose. Never use less than half a tablet. You should note that capsules and enteric-coated medications cannot be crushed or broken.

Manually-controlled infusions

The infusion rate equals the 'volume' (in drops) divided by 'time' (in minutes). To be able to calculate the rate, you will need to know how many drops per millilitre the administration set delivers. This information can usually be found on the bag.

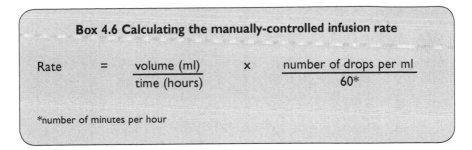

Box 4.6 Calculating the manually-controlled infusion rate

Rate = $\dfrac{\text{volume (ml)}}{\text{time (hours)}}$ x $\dfrac{\text{number of drops per ml}}{60^*}$

*number of minutes per hour

However, a general guide is:

- Clear fluids = 20 drops/ml
- Blood = 15 drops/ml

For example, 1 litre of normal saline (clear fluid) to be administered over 6 hours:

Rate = $\dfrac{1000}{6}$ x $\dfrac{20}{60}$ = $\dfrac{20000}{360}$ = $\dfrac{500}{9}$ = 55.55 = 56 drops per minute

Mechanically-controlled infusion

Mechanically-controlled infusion uses a volumetric pump. This apparatus requires that you set the correct infusion rate, measured in ml per hour:

Rate = $\dfrac{\text{volume (ml)}}{\text{time (hours)}}$ = $\dfrac{\text{volume (ml)}}{\text{time (minutes)}}$ x 60

For example, 1 litre of normal saline over 6 hours:

Rate = $\dfrac{1000}{6}$ = 166.66 = 167ml per hour

However, there may be occasions where small amounts have to be administered. Antibiotics, for example, are sometimes given over 20 minutes, half an hour or 100 minutes. Administering 250ml over 100 minutes:

Rate = $\dfrac{250}{100}$ x 60 = 150 ml per hour

Some practice calculations

Try the following calculations, without a calculator to begin with (answers are available at the end of the chapter).

1) Multiply:
   (a) 83 x 10
   (b) 03 A 100
   (c) 83 x 1000

2) Multiply:
   (a) 0.0258 x 10
   (b) 0.0258 x 100
   (c) 0.0258 x 1000

3) Divide:
   (a) 3.78 ÷ 10
   (b) 3.78 ÷ 100
   (c) 3.78 ÷ 1000

4) Change:
   (a) 0.78 grams to milligrams
   (b) 34 milligrams to grams
   (c) 0.086 milligrams to micrograms
   (d) 294 micrograms to milligrams
   (e) 2.4 litres to millilitres
   (f) 965 millilitres to litres

Drug doses for injection

1) An injection of 8mg of morphine is required. The ampoule contains 10mg in 1ml. What volume should be drawn up for injection?
2) An injection of erythromycin 120mg is prescribed. The stock vials contain 300mg/10ml. What volume is required
3) A labouring woman of small build is to be given 75mg of pethidine. The ampoule is 100mg/2ml what volume is required?
4) A neonate is prescribed 1mg of phytomenadione. The vial contain 2mg in 0.2ml. What volume is required?

Doses of oral medication

Calculate the oral doses to be given of the following:

1) Ranitidine 225mg orally is ordered. Syrup that has 75mg in 5ml is available.
2) Cephalexin 500mg four times a day is required. How many tablets will the woman need to take home for a seven day course.
3) Ampicillin syrup 500mg is ordered. Syrup of 125mg in 5ml is available.
4) Eythromycin 800mg is ordered. Syrup of 125mg in 5ml is available.

Infusion rates

Calculate the drops per minute:

1) 800ml Hartmann's solution is to be infused over 10 hours. The IV set delivers 15 drops/ml.
2) 325ml blood is to be given over 4 hours. The IV set delivers 15 drops/ml.
3) 800ml of fluid is to drip at 50 drops/min. How long will the fluid last if the IV set delivers 15 drops/ml?
4) Half a litre of fluid is to be given at 25 drops/min The IV set delivers 15 drops/ml. How long will it take to deliver this amount?

Some final calculations:

How can I calculate the the mean arterial pressure (MAP)?

The mean arterial pressure (MAP) can be calculated as follows:

MAP = diastolic blood pressure (BP) + 1/3(systolic BP – diastolic BP)

For example, calculating the MAP when the blood pressure is 160/100:

MAP = 100 + 1/3(160-100)
100 + 1/3(60)
100 + 20
120mmHg

How can I calculate the body mass index (BMI)?

$$BMI = \frac{\text{weight (kg)}}{[\text{height (m)}]^2}$$

Normal range: 20–25
Underweight: <20
Overweight: 25.1–30
Obese: >30

How can I avoid drug errors?

Annie Law/Jacqui Williams

It is worth bearing in mind that administering drugs in a busy ward can be rather like driving a car, in that it is easy to allow a sense of routine to take over and not concentrate fully on the job in hand. Like driving, mistakes can happen at any time, and they may prove fatal.'

(Nursing Times 1994)

There are two main types of error:
- **Error of omission** — where the midwife unintentionally fails to administer a prescribed drug.
- **Error of commission** — where the midwife administers a drug that was not prescribed, or gives an excessive dose of a prescribed drug.

(adapted from Nursing Times 1994)

In the past, drug errors have been linked with blame and would often lead to disciplinary action. This led to fear of reporting errors potential harm to women (DoH 2000). Today the NHS promotes an 'open, no blame' culture, which encourages reporting. However, all incidents require a thorough investigation to be able to distinguish between errors that:

- Were concealed.
- Occurred as a result of reckless or in competence practice,
- Occurred as a result of pressure of work.
- Were immediately and honestly disclosed.

(NMC 2008)

The National Patient Safety Agency (NPSA) has been charged with the task of ensuring that error reports and the lessons learned from them are disseminated throughout the NHS (Shepherd 2002).

Risk management strategies use 'near misses' as a way of reducing systemic errors by ensuring that sufficient information is available to prescribers, by promoting electronic prescribing to reduce the risk of errors form poor handwriting and by integrating pharmacists into clinical teams, to anticipate errors rather than discover them (Audit Commission 2001; Cavell and Hughes 1997).

Lack of knowledge is a common cause of error (Cavell 2000) and when there are two women with the same name, you must be particularly vigilant. Make sure you are familiar with the 2007 NMC's Standards for Medicine Management as well as your own Trust guidelines.

References

Audit Commission (2001) *A Spoonful of Sugar: medicines management in NHS hospitals.* London, Audit Commission.

Bainbridge L, Nasmith MD, Orchard C, Wood V (2010) Competencies for interprofessional collaboration. *Journal of Physical Therapy Education.* **24(1):** 6-11. Available from www.ipe.uwo.ca (accessed 17/7/11)

Dulin Y, Bodian C, Weiser J et al (2005) Anesthesiology: Pain and Regional Anesthesia. **103** http://journals.lww.com/anesthesiology//abstract/2005/12000/Effect_of_Labor_Epidural_Analgesia_with_and.16.aspx (accessed 10/3/11)

Bragg F, Cromwell D, Edozien L, Gurol-Urganci I, Mahmood T, Templeton,A, Van der Meulan J (2010) Variations in rates of caesarean section among NHS trusts after accounting of maternal and clinical risk: cross-sectional study. *BMJ.* **341:** c5065 www.bjm.com (accessed 1/3/11)

Carne V (2009) Epidurals in labour. *Essence Midwifery Newsletter* p1-4 www.midirs.com

Cavell G (2000) Drugs: the nurses' responsibility. *Professional Nurse.* **15(5):** 296

Cavell G, Hughes DK (1997) Does computerised prescribing improve the accuracy of drug administration? *Pharmaceutical Journal* **259:** 782-4

Department of Health (1998) *The new NHS, modern and dependable: A national framework for assessing performance.* Stationery Office, London.

Department of Health (2000) *The NHS Plan: a plan for investment, a plan for reform.* Stationery Office, London.

Department of Health (2000) *An organisation with a memory: report of an expert group on learning from adverse events in the NHS.* Stationery Office, London.

Department of Health (2008) *A high quality workforce: NHS next stage review.* Stationery Office, London.

Devroe S, Decoster, Van De Velde (2009) Breastfeeding and epidural analgesic during labour. *Opinion in Anaesthesiology* **22(3):** 327-9

Dimond B (2004) *Legal Aspects of Nursing. 4th edn.* Longman, New York.

Homeyard C, Forrester M (2011) Midwives exemptions. *Essentially MIDIRS.* **2(4):** 32-36

Lavender T, Kingdon C (2006) Keeping birth normal. In Page LA, McCandlish R (Eds) *The new midwifery: science and sensitivity in practice. 2nd edn.* Churchill-Livingstone, Edinburgh.

Lowden G (1995a) Of no consequence. www.casearean.org.uk/articles/OfNoCons.html (accessed 7/1/11)

Lowden G (1995b) Actually. www.casearean.org.uk/articles/Actually.html (accessed 7/1/11)

Midwifery 2020 Programme (2010) Midwifery 2020 delivery expectations September. www.midwifery2020.org (accessed 5/1/11)

National Health Service Litigation Authority (2010) Clinical Negligence Scheme for Trusts Maternity Clinical Risk Management Standards 2011/12. www.nhlsa.com

National Prescribing Centre (2009) September. www.npc.co.uk (accessed 5/1/11)

National Institute for Health and Clinical Excellence (2004) Caesarean Section London. NICE www.nice.org.uk

Newburn M, Dodds R (2010) Breastfeeding support, active listening and guidance during matrescence. *Essentially MIDIRS* **1(1):** 32-6

Nursing and Midwifery Council (NMC) (2009) *Supply and/or administration of medicine by student nurses and student midwives in relation to Patient Group Directions (PGDs).* NMC, London.

Nursing and Midwifery Council (NMC) (2007) *Standards for medicines management.* NMC, London.

Nursing and Midwifery Council (NMC) (2004) *Midwives Rules and Standards* NMC, London

Nursing Times (1994) Professional development, medication: the role of the nurse. *Nurs Times.* **90(37 suppl.):** 5-8

Reynolds F (2010) The effect of maternal labour analgesia on the fetus. *Best Pract Res Clin Obstet Gynaecol* **24(3):** 289-302

World Health Organisation (1996) *Care in normal birth: a practical guide.* WHO, Geneva

Answers

Practice calculations
1) (a) 830; (b) 8300; (c) 83000
2) (a) 0.258; (b) 2.58; (c) 25.8;
3) (a) 0.378; (b) 0.0378; (c) 0.00378
4) (a) 780mg; (b) 0.034g; (c) 86000µg; (d) 0.294mg; (e) 2400ml; (f) 0.965l

Drug doses for injection
1) 0.8ml; 2) 4ml; 3) 1.5ml; 4) 0.1ml

Doses of oral medication
1) 15ml; 2) 28ml; 3) 20ml; 4) 32ml

Infusion rates
1) 20 drops/min; 2) 20 drops/min; 3) 4 hours; 4) 5 hours

Chapter 5: Dealing with challenging situations

- **What is my role in the care of the obese childbearing woman?**
- **How do I give appropriate care to new parents who have a disability?**
- **What are the issues in caring for childbearing women from ethnic minority backgrounds?**
- **What is my role in clinical emergencies?**
- **How do I deal with a shoulder dystocia?**
- **How do I deal with a postpartum haemorrhage?**
- **How do I deal with a cord prolapse?**
- **What do I do if I find an undiagnosed breech in labour?**

What is my role in the care of the obese childbearing woman?

Rowena Doughty

In 2008, according to the body mass index (BMI) classification, 20.2% of women of childbearing age (aged 16–44) in the UK were obese (BMI≥30) (NOO 2010; Cullum 2009; Heslehurst *et al* 2007; Kanagalingam *et al* 2005). Risk factors for obesity in the pregnant population include increasing age, increasing parity and social deprivation (NOO 2010), although the demographic characteristics of the pregnant population appear similar to those of the non-pregnant population.

Obesity is one of the most significant health concerns in our society. A number of disease pathways are attributable to obesity, including cardiovascular disease, certain cancers and type 2 diabetes (WHO 2005) and an individual's risk of serious morbidity and/or mortality is directly related to increasing body weight.

Therefore, obesity has a significant influence on pregnancy outcomes. It has been reported as a factor in 35% of maternal deaths (Lewis 2007) and the trend in the rate of obesity is upward one. According to one study, an estimated 50% of women of childbearing age will be obese by 2050 (Foresight 2007).

What causes obesity and how is it diagnosed?

Obesity is caused by the excessive accumulation of fat within adipocytes, resulting from a discrepancy between energy intake and energy expenditure. It is diagnosed using the BMI classification.

BMI is calculated by dividing the body weight in kilograms by the square of the height in metres. Where BMI is equal to or greater than 30, a person is classified as 'obese'. This classification can be further subdivided — where BMI is equal to or greater than 40, the person is classified as having 'extreme obesity'. However, the distribution of body fat is also significant — an increased waist to hip ratio is thought to be more important than increased weight alone, and disordered glucose tolerance is likely to be found on testing (WHO 2002).

What are the risks associated with obesity in childbearing women?

- **Infertility** — Polycystic Ovary Syndrome (PCOS) is associated with obesity, and can have a negative influence on fertility.
- **Early miscarriage** — both early and recurrent miscarriage have been shown to have associations with obesity.
- **Congenital abnormality (e.g. neural tube defects [NTD']s)** — it can be argued that congenital abnormalities are more likely to occur as ultrasound visualisation is poorer and there is also a higher incidence of diabetes in obese women, which is associated with congenital abnormality.
- **Presence of comorbidities** — obesity increases the risks of conditions such as type 2 diabetes, acquired cardiac disease and hypertension, which all have a negative influence on maternal mortality and morbidity and pregnancy outcomes.
- **Macrosomia** — birth weights of greater than 4kg are associated with maternal obesity and can lead to problems during birth e.g. shoulder dystocia.
- **Intra-uterine fetal death/stillbirth** — late fetal death is associated with obesity, especially in first-time mums.
- **Gestational diabetes:** carbohydrate intolerance and insulin resistance is seen more commonly as BMI increases, making gestational diabetes more common in obese women.
- **Pregnancy-induced hypertension (PIH)** — essential hypertension is more common in obese women. Superimposed PIH and pre-eclamptic toxaemia (PET) may develop, and these carry additional risks. Obese women with associated hypertension are more likely to have small for gestational age babies.

- **Venous thromboembolism (VTE)** — pregnancy creates a 'hypercoagulable state' to minimise haemorrhage, and this increases the risk of VTE. The risk is further increased in women with obesity — it is unclear why, but increased sedentary lifestyles may be a factor.
- **Prolonged pregnancy** — this increases the incidence of induction of labour and its associated problems.
- **Operative birth** — prolonged labour is often seen in obese women, which increases the incidence of operative birth. Obesity increases anaesthetic, perioperative and postpartum risks, and decreases the likelihood of success-ful vaginal birth after caesarean (VBAC).
- **Postnatal Complications (e.g. postpartum haemorrhage)** — wound infections are more common in obese women following operative birth.
- **Difficulties with breastfeeding** — fewer obese women successfully breastfeed. The reasons are multi-faceted but include delayed lactogenesis, a slow milk ejection reflex and they may receive poorer advice on positioning and attachment etc.
- **Perinatal mental health** — obese individuals often experience stigma and discrimination associated with their weight, which can lead to low self-esteem and confidence, which is associated with increased rates of depression.

What is the role of the midwife?

Antenatal

- Calculate the woman's BMI as part of the 'booking' interview. Women with a BMI ≥30 should be referred to a consultant for shared care.
- Consider continuity of midwifery support to improve self-esteem and self-confidence.
- Consider VTE prophylaxis.
- Ensure that all women with a BMI ≥40 take a vitamin D supplement.
- Women should book to birth in a consultant-led environment.
- Refer women to other agencies e.g. dietetics.
- Screen all women with a BMI ≥30 for gestational diabetes and repeat glu-cose tolerance testing (GTT) at six weeks postnatal.
- Refer women to a specialist team if they have a BMI ≥35 and another significant risk factor (such as smoking, multiple pregnancy) as they are at risk of PIH and PET.
- Offer additional antenatal appointments — every three weeks from 24–32 weeks and then fortnightly from 32 weeks until birth.
- Encourage women to attend antenatal preparation classes.

- Advise women to monitor their weight gain in pregnancy and ensure it is not excessive.
- Dieting in pregnancy is not recommended, but provide all women with individually-tailored advice about healthy eating.
- Give specific advice on screening options and explain how being overweight can affect test results.
- Throughout pregnancy, carefully observe maternal and fetal status, to detect any complications.
- Perform a risk assessment for the birth — are there any moving and handling considerations? What care is needed to preserve tissue viability?
- Ensure a multidisciplinary birth plan has been created for all women with a BMI ≥30.
- Refer all women with a BMI ≥40 to an anaesthetist.
- Communicate effectively with the multidisciplinary team (MDT), your manager and your Supervisor of Midwives, as appropriate.

Intrapartum

- Provide effective midwifery support during labour. All women with a BMI ≥40 should have one-to-one support.
- Ensure that you read and communicate the plan of care.
- Inform the anesthetist if a woman with a BMI ≥40 is admitted in labour.
- Encourage women to remain mobile and to change position regularly, avoiding supine positions and promoting upright positions, to utilise gravity.
- Ensure that women avoid dehydration during labour, as this increases the risk of VTE.
- Ensure that all the equipment you use is suitable for the woman e.g. large BP cuff, bed that will support her weight.
- Effectively use the partogram to observe progress in labour.
- Consider attaching a fetal scalp electrode (FSE) if you are unable to adequately auscultate the fetal heart trans-abdominally.
- Be vigilant for complications, e.g. signs of impending shoulder dystocia
- Management of the third stage — active management is recommended and you should secure venous access.

Postnatal

- Liaise closely with the anaesthetist — these women may require increased analgesia postnatally.
- Encourage the woman to mobilise as soon as possible and continue thrombo-embolic prophylaxis until she is fully mobile, to reduce the risk of VTE.

- Inform the woman about delayed lactogenesis and tailor breastfeeding advice. For example, women with larger breasts may find the underarm method more effective when positioning the neonate at the breast.
- Consider giving advice on contraception. Some types of contraception may be contra-indicated due to women's weight or the presence of underlying medical conditions.
- Observe closely for signs of postnatal depression.
- Consider referral to other agencies e.g. dietetics, psychotherapy.
- Women may benefit from extended postnatal midwifery care.
- Handover the woman's care directly to her GP and the health visitor, making sure that both are aware of her postnatal BMI, so they can follow-up for sustained weight loss management.

How do I give appropriate care to new parents who have a disability?

Bernadette Gregory

The legal definition of disability is:

'A physical or mental impairment which has substantial and long term adverse effects on a person's ability to perform normal day to day activities.'
(www.direct.gov.uk 2011)

Only 17% of disabled people are born with their impairment (RCN 2007). Disabilities can be acquired through injury, accidents, disease or as a result of increasing age — anyone can become disabled at any time, regardless of gender, age, sexual orientation, religion or race. The Disability Discrimination Act (DDA) also includes progressive conditions, such as cancer, HIV infection and multiple sclerosis, which can affect an individual's abilities in the future.

The Equality Act (2010) brings together previous legislation and reminds midwives and service providers that we are all personally and professionally responsible for ensuring that services and information are available to all parents.

The issues of 'who is disabled?' and 'what is disability?' are more complex than mere legal definitions. For one thing, it is difficult to determine accurate data. Benefit uptake dates are unreliable — the Royal College of Nursing (RCN) (2007) has suggested that of the 10.8 million people in the UK who identify themselves as 'disabled', approximately 52% of those who qualify for benefits do not claim them.

Data from the RCN (2007) suggests that:

- 4 million people have physical impairments.
- 5% of the disabled population are wheelchair users.
- 2 million have visual impairments.
- 3.5 million have a hearing impairment.
- 62,000 use British Sign Language (BSL) as their preferred language.
- 1.5 million people have learning disabilities.
- 8.6 million have long-term mental health problems (RCN 2007).

Additional barriers for parents living with a disability

'While the majority of non-disabled parents can take it for granted that the quality and character of their parenting is their own business ... disabled women really do feel under surveillance, and that feeling is usually well-founded because disabled women are assumed by professionals and lay people (often including close relatives) to be incapable unless they can prove otherwise: guilty until proven innocent.'

(Thomas 1997)

It is not only health professionals that judge whether parents living with a disability are competent but also family members. Thomas (1997) states that in her research involving 17 women, accounts 'testify to the particular vulnerability that many women with impairments feel when they become mothers'. So, what can you do to provide the additional support that these people need in their new role as parents?

A number of parents and health professionals have worked together to develop networks for information, resources and publications — some local and some national. Where one or both parents have a disability, there may be concerns over how they will cope. You must remember that they are the experts when it comes to their disabilities and they may seek help at an early stage of pregnancy. They will expect health professionals to be able to organise appropriate additional help and specialist support.

Midwives need to be aware of the additional support and monies parents can access, and must adopt a multi-agency approach to care needs.

Although McKay and Moffatt's study (2007) involved only eight midwives from three maternity units, they found that midwives had positive attitudes to parents living with disabilities, using phrases such as 'the mother's advocate' and

Box 5.1 Pause for thought

Do you know the answers to the following questions?

A woman with a hearing impairment asks:

> *"How will I know when the baby wakes up? Are there special alarms to buy?"*
> *"Can I attend parent craft classes- is there a LOOP system in that building?"*

A wheelchair user asks:

> *"Is there a lift or ramp access for my wheelchair?"*
> *"Where are the nearest Blue Badge car park spaces?"*

A woman with a visual impairment asks:

> *"Can I bring my guide dog into hospital with me?"*

'working in partnership'. They found that all the midwives thought individual women with disabilities 'should be treated the same as every woman, without her disability being paramount' and also that they felt they 'lacked knowledge and experience in some aspects of care provision'.

Some mothers in the same study raised concerns about midwives' lack of knowledge of their conditions. For example, a mother with multiple sclerosis 'felt that the midwives lacked understanding about her condition', which resulted in 'insensitive and intolerant care and failure to give her prescribed medication regularly'. However, four other mothers experienced care that was 'sensitive, respectful and responsive to their needs while maintaining their privacy and dignity, which they valued' and which 'contributed to feelings of satisfaction with their care'. Lipson and Rogers (2000) noted that people with less visible disabilities 'often receive insensitive care' (cited in McKay and Cunningham 2007).

Midwives are now more involved in the multidisciplinary approach to care

(NMC 2004) and are able to visit longer into the postnatal period. The public health agenda means that midwives are at the front line of assessing parental competence (O'Luanaigh 2004; National Parenting Institute 2007). This is crucial for caring for women living with disability.

The Royal College of Obstetricians and Gynaecologists' (RCOG) 'Standards for Maternity Care' (2008) state that:

- Each maternity service should have an explicit plan for antenatal care for all women.
- A system of clear referral paths should be established.
- All women should be able to contact a midwife day or night at any stage in pregnancy if they have concerns.

(RCOG 2008)

Key practice points

- You must become familiar with the useful resources list below to help parents living with a disability fulfil their parenting roles.
- Consider how accessible your practice area is to parents living with disabilities and where possible, make appropriate changes.
- You should make provisions for parents living with disabilities, e.g. at parent education classes, antenatal clinics, when they are on the postnatal ward.

Useful resources

The following organisations promote good practice and provide resources that raise awareness of the additional support that parents with disabilities may need:

Disability, Pregnancy and Parenthood International
The UK's national information charity on disability and parenthood.
www.dppi.org.uk

Royal National Institute for the Deaf
http://www.actiononhearingloss.org.uk/

Royal National Institute for the Blind
www.rnib.org.uk

National Childbirth Trust

The UK's largest charity for parents.

www.nct.org.uk

CHANGE

A leading national human rights organisation led by people with learning disabilities.

www.changepeople.co.uk

Ann Craft Trust

A national charity working with professionals, parents, carers to protect children and adults with learning disabilities from abuse.

www.anncrafttrust.org

What are the issues in caring for childbearing women from ethnic minority backgrounds?

Zaheera Essat

British society is multicultural and its diversity of beliefs and practices cannot be overlooked (Raphael-Leff 1991). It is during the transition to motherhood that women are at their most vulnerable and sensitive, and the quality of care and support they receive affects their ability to cope (Schott and Henley 1996). Midwives care for women from many diverse cultures and backgrounds, some of whom will have migrated from other countries. To ensure a positive childbearing experience, it is important that ethnic minority women receive care that is appropriate to their needs (Jackson 1994).

Women who migrate to Britain are often marginalised. They lack support systems that other women may have to cope with the transition to motherhood and birth in an environment that is not within their context (Raphael-Leff 1991). In a western industrial society, the context of childbearing is based on a medical model. However, this concept is unfamiliar to migrant women from societies that advocate the traditional management of birth (Katbamna 2000). Through traditional practices, birth is reinforced as a social act, connecting women within a community (Kitzinger, 2000).

A misconception that midwives commonly have, is that all ethnic minorities are part of one group, so universal care is appropriate with the help of a 'cultural recipe book' (Bowler 1993). Women who belong to ethnic, cultural and religious groups are often grouped together and their way of life is compared with a 'standard white model', which is seen as ideal (Smart and Shipman 2004). Health professionals must challenge their assumptions and listen to these women (Holloway and Wheeler 2002). The actions of ethnic minorities are often compared with those of indigenous groups, and seen as 'different' rather than 'diverse' (Berthoud 2000). Those who cannot embrace a multi-ethnic society see migrants as 'traditional and unchangeable' (Zontini 2007). However, the indigenous population is itself incredibly diverse, and host to a wide range of different values (Berthoud 2000).

The beliefs and values of migrants are often categorised using binaries such as 'ethnic/mainstream' or 'traditional/modern' (Zonitini 2000). Ethnic minority families are commonly categorised as holding 'old-fashioned' rather than 'modern-individualistic' values (Berthoud 2000). However, ethnic minority families in Britain are constantly changing and 'tradition' itself 'is something under constant change and negotiation' (Smart and Shipman 2004). Many migrant families are comfortable with adopting both traditional and modern practices — individualisation does not necessarily equate to the abandonment of traditional practices (Smart and Shipman 2004; Essat 2010).

The reality is that midwives are working in a system that has limited resources, which makes it very difficult to meet women's needs. However, even small and inexpensive changes can be effective. Research suggests that the support that women give each other has positive effects on childbearing, both physically and emotionally (Hall 2001). Women who give birth in Britain are likely to build a connecting relationship with their midwife, who will often take over the supportive role, replacing family members who are not there physically (Laryea 1989; Silverton 1993). The midwife's role will ensure that the woman's needs are met (Hall 2001). Midwives who offer continuity of care are likely to achieve a connecting relationship with the women they care for (Sandall 1997). Many midwives use a bio-psychosocial model, wherein 'individuals are viewed holistically and within their context — family, community and culture' (Barnett, Matthey and Boyce 1999). A woman's ability to birth and recuperate can amaze even an experienced midwife.

What is my role in clinical emergencies?

You must be fully conversant with emergency drills and take every opportunity to practice them, so that you can act promptly and efficiently when an emergency arises. The question of who should take charge in a clinical emergency is largely supported by anecdotal evidence, which suggests that allied health professionals should defer to their medical colleagues. However, midwives must be fully informed about their responsibilities and sphere of practice, and must ensure that the most appropriate health professional is called when there is deviation from the norm (NMC 2004). The midwife may be the most appropriate person to be team leader in an emergency, but she must ensure that a more senior obstetrician is referred to.

How do I deal with shoulder dystocia?

Rowena Doughty/Jacqui Williams

Shoulder dystocia is an obstetric emergency that occurs in roughly 1 in 200 births (RCOG 2005). As well as threatening the fetus, it causes an increase in maternal morbidity, with the rate of postpartum haemorrhage rising to 11%. To reduce risks to both the woman and the fetus, it is important to recognise what is happening and to promptly commence the drill.

The HELPERRS mnemonic is a useful tool to guide practice. Box 5.2 overleaf details the HELPERRS mnemonic and midwife's role during shoulder dystocia.

How do I deal with a postpartum haemorrhage (PPH)?

Bernadette Gregory/Jacqui Williams

Definition

An excessive bleeding from the genital tract occurring at any time from the birth of the child to 12 weeks postnatal.

What is a primary PPH?

The commonest PPH and the most dangerous (Mousa and Alfiric 2007), occurring within the first 24 hours. Its incidence is approximately 6% of all deliveries.

Box 5.2 The HELPERRS mnemonic for the management of shoulder dystocia

H **Call for Help** — note the time of delivery of the fetal head. Recognise the emergency and take control of the situation. If in unit, pull the emergency buzzer to summon assistance, or dial 999 if in the community. Briefly inform the woman of the situation and ask for her co-operation. Ask her to stop pushing, or this will further impact the anterior shoulder. Auscultate the fetal heart if possible.

E **Evaluate for Episiotomy** — only really useful if performing internal manoeuvres; remember that this is a bony problem, not a soft tissue problem.

L **McRoberts' position – Legs** — lie the woman flat with her knees/legs extended, then legs bent and drawn up towards her chest. This position rotates the symphysis pubis (SP) superiorly, relieving pressure on the SP by the fetal shoulder; it elevates the anterior shoulder, flexes the fetal spine, straightens maternal lordosis and opens the pelvic inlet/outlet — attempt normal traction for 30-60 seconds.

P **Suprapubic Pressure** — continuous or rocking movement performed over the fetal back by a second midwife — this reduces the bisacromial diameter and encourages the anterior shoulder into an oblique diameter (external Rubins'/Rubins' I). Can be used with all internal manoeuvres — if used with McRoberts', this is successful in 60–80% of cases. Once the anterior shoulder is free, perform downward traction to deliver the baby.

E **Enter to perform internal manoeuvres** — perform an episiotomy if now possible. Undertake internal manoeuvres with the woman in McRoberts' position (with SP pressure) or in an 'all fours' position. No specific order is recommended:

1. Perform Woods' manoeuvre:
   - Insert two fingers into the vagina and locate the anterior surface of the posterior shoulder over the clavicle
   - The posterior shoulder is then rotated 180° in the direction of the fetal back with supra-pubic pressure, which disimpacts the anterior shoulder and allows the posterior shoulder to enter the pelvic brim
   - The posterior shoulder, which is now the anterior shoulder, may now be delivered by normal manoeuvres.

Rowena Doughty ©2009

2. Perform Rubins' II manoeuvre:
- The midwife's hand is inserted into the vagina to locate the posterior aspect of the anterior shoulder
The shoulders are then pushed from behind into an oblique diameter, which adducts the shoulders and reduces the bisacromial diameter
- The shoulders are then free of the symphysis pubis and delivery can be completed.
n.b. Woods' and Rubins' II can be performed together, if possible.
If unsuccessful:
3. Perform reverse Woods' manoeuvre:
- The fingers that were behind the anterior shoulder are moved down to the posterior aspect of the posterior shoulder
- Attempt to rotate the fetus 180° in the opposite direction, to deliver the fetus.

R **Remove of the posterior arm** — removal of the posterior arm:
- Insert the hand into the vagina, along the curve of the sacrum, and locate the posterior arm — antecubital pressure will flex the elbow
- Sweep this arm across the chest and deliver it — the fetus should then deliver spontaneously with downward traction as diameters are reduced
- This is often considered before the other internal manoeuvres, especially if woman is in the 'all fours' position.

R **Roll over onto 'all-fours'** — this may be used before trying internal manoeuvres and it may be easier to perform internal manoeuvres with the woman in this position. This is considered to be an upside-down McRoberts — it is useful in minor cases, but supra-pubic pressure cannot be used as effectively. Consider a change of position in mobile women (>80% success rate) but beware in women with epidural analgesia, or those who are tired or uncooperative. It may be useful in women who are obese.

S **Start all over again** — each procedure should be undertaken for 20–30 seconds before moving on to the next. If nothing works, return to the beginning and start again.

Post event — be prepared to resuscitate the baby and take cord gases. Also, be prepared for a possible postpartum haemorrhage and repair any perineal trauma. Fully document the event in the patient records and complete a risk management form. Debrief parents and seek the support of your Supervisor of Midwives.

What is a secondary PPH?

This occurs after 24 hours and up to 12 weeks postnatal (Alexander *et al* 2002). The incidence is 1–3% of all pregnancies.

- A PPH is traditionally more than 500ml (WHO 1990; 1989).
- Smaller losses than this are treated as serious, later in the puerperium.
- Definitions are of limited value — it is much more important to assess the effects of blood loss on the mother.
- In some contexts, 'excessive' may be a much smaller amount, which may affect the mother.

How is blood loss defined?

- Minor: 500–1000ml
- Major: >1000ml
  - Moderate: 1000–2000ml
  - Severe: >2000ml

(RCOG 2009)

Estimating blood loss — how scientific is it?

- It is difficult to measure.
- It is unreliable.
- It is often underestimated.
- It is unpredictable.
- It can be unexpected.

(Levy and Moore 1985; Prasertcharoensuk et al 2000;
Buckland and Homer 2007)

What are the causes of a PPH?

- The placental site.
- Failure of the uterus to adequately contract and retract.
- A flaccid or atonic myometrium.
- Retained products.
- Genital tract trauma/damage (cervical, vaginal or uterine?)

What risk factors should I consider?

- History of previous PPH or retained placenta and membranes.
- A multiple pregnancy.
- Polyhydramnios.
- Anaemia in pregnancy.
- Antepartum haemorrhage (APH).
- Prolonged labour.
- Pre-eclampsia/pregnancy-induced hypertension (PIH).
- General anaesthesia.
- Fibroids.
- Mismanagement of the 3rd stage of labour.
- Retained placenta or retained products.
- Tocolytic drugs.
- Induced or augmented labour.
- Inversion of the uterus.
- Infection, e.g. chorioamnionitis.
- Grande multiparity.
- Disseminating Intravascular Coagulation (DIC).
- Clotting disorders.
- Unknown.

Prevention is better than cure

- **Preconception** — optimal health to begin pregnancy, correct any anaemia.
- **Pregnancy** — identify risk factors, diagnose and treat anaemia.
- **Labour** — policy guidelines, good management during 1st, 2nd and 3rd stages of labour — treat the uterus with respect!
- Active management of 3rd stage (RCOG 2009)
- **After delivery** — careful monitoring for the first hour postnatal

What are the principles of good management?

- Assessment.
- Stop any bleeding.
- Resuscitation.
- Fluid replacement.
- Hospitalisation.

What if you are at the woman's home?

* Call the paramedic team to attend.
* Take blood for cross-matching, full blood count (FBC), clotting studies and site a large bore canula — start fluids.
* Take and record vital signs.
* Keep all evidence of blood loss.
* Inform an appropriate person at the referring delivery suite and give an accurate account of the woman's condition.
* Arrange transfer to hospital as soon as possible.
* Travel with the woman and during transfer, monitor her condition and give oxygen.

What are the principles of care?

* Ascertain the site of the bleeding.
* Deliver the placenta and membranes.
* 'Rub up a contraction'.
* Give an oxytocic drug — syntometrine and/or ergometrine.
* Monitor vital signs frequently.
* Empty her bladder.
* Prepare for theatre — intravenous fluids and order blood.
* Manually remove the placenta and membranes.

After delivery of the placenta and membranes

* 'Rub up a contraction'.
* Give an oxytocic drug.
* If necessary, empty the bladder.

If the midwife suspects that the uterus is not well-contracted and there is excessive blood loss, it is essential that these steps are taken as soon as possible:

* Check the placenta and membranes for completeness.
* Arrange theatre for evacuation of any retained products of conception.

How do you do external manual compression?

The left hand dips down as far as possible behind the uterus. The right hand is pressed flat on the abdominal wall; the uterus is compressed and pulled upwards into the abdomen.

When is internal bimanual compression used?

- It is carried out under general anaesthetic.
- The right hand is inserted into the vagina, closed to form a fist and pushed up in direction of the anterior vaginal fornix. The left hand is placed on the vaginal wall, dips down behind the uterus, pulls it forwards and towards the symphysis pubis. Both hands are pressed firmly together, compressing the uterus and placental site. Continue pressure until the uterus contracts and remains retracted.

What is abdominal aortic compression?

A short-term emergency measure while awaiting emergency assistance. The midwife places a fist on the mother's abdomen, above the fundus and below the level of the renal arteries (L1/2).

Could the PPH be due to trauma?

Approximately 20% of cases of PPH arise from a laceration of some part of the genital tract (Llewellyn Jones 1999).

Treatment may be:

- Direct pressure.
- Application of sponge forceps.
- Suturing under GA or regional anaesthetic.
- If there is a tear on the uterus, the woman may need a hysterectomy.
- Vulval haematoma may occur.

Maternal effects

- Anaemia.
- Blood-coagulation disorders including DIC.
- Widespread tissue damage:
  - Renal — oliguria or anuria
  - Cardiac failure
    Respiratory failure
  - Liver damage — jaundice
  - Brain damage — convulsions and coma
  - Pituitary gland involvement — Sheehan's syndrome.
- Maternal mortality and morbidity.

Massive obstetric haemorrhage (MOH) — confidential enquiries

Recurrent themes:

- Failure to recognise problems.
- Failure to take action.
- Failure to refer.
- Inappropriate delegation.
- Lack of team work.

50% of maternal deaths and 75% of intrapartum deaths are potentially avoidable.

Maternal Deaths 2000–2002

Substandard clinical care led to:

- Failure to recognise and act on common signs of critical illness.
- Lack of follow-up of non-attenders.
- Failure to communicate relevant medical history.
- Poor communication and team working in multidisciplinary teams (MDT)
- Failure to call early for senior help.
- Wrong diagnosis or treatment.

Recommendations:

- Skills drills to improve the management of MOH.
- Teamwork training.
- Take a multi-professional approach.
- Protocols for MOH involving blood bank (SML 2003–2005).
- Annual multi-professional training for all staff (NHS 2010).

How do I deal with a cord prolapse?

Jacqui Williams

Your role demands that you promptly recognise when the cord has prolapsed and take appropriate action. You must ask yourself the following key questions:

- What is the fetal condition?
- What is the cervical dilatation?

What action should you take? An instrumental delivery may be feasible, or if possible within 15 minutes, an emergency caesarean section may be an option. If the fetus is not alive, spontaneous delivery will be awaited.

Recommended actions:

- Call for assistance.
- Note the time.
- Position the woman knee-chest (exaggerated Sims' position).
- Apply digital pressure to the presenting part, to keep the weight off cord.
- Monitor the fetal heart rate throughout.
- Consider filling the bladder via a Foley catheter with 150ml normal saline.
- Give ranitidine 150mg and prepare for delivery/theatre.
- Reassure the woman and her partner promptly and communicate the situation so they can cooperate with your requests.
- Transfer to theatre/from the community in the supine position, with a wedge (due to safety issues).
- Documentation — record all events and actions.
- Prepare for resuscitation of the baby, ensure that the paediatrician/ neonatologist has been called, take cord bloods.
- Following the delivery, sensitively debrief the woman and her partner.
- Complete an incident form and ensure that you are debriefed yourself, possibly with your Supervisor of Midwives.

What do I do if I find an undiagnosed breech in labour?

Jacqui Williams

At 28 weeks' gestation, 20% of fetuses will be presenting breech — by term, this reduces to 3–4% (RCOG 2006). Penn (2006) proposes that 10% of breech presentations will not be identified before term and you need to be mindful of this when you first meet the woman in labour.

If breech is suspected in labour, you must urgently seek appropriate medical help. An experienced obstetrician is needed, as a safe vaginal delivery may be possible (RCOG 2006). Do not rely on previous palpations and vaginal examinations as they may not be accurate and the fetal position may have changed.

The following points will need to be considered to ensure that the safest mode of delivery can be determined:

- Parity.
- Gestation.
- Past obstetric history.
- Presentation — absence of footling breech.
- Fetal weight (estimate).
- Clinical assessment of pelvic size.
- The woman and her partner's wishes, after careful discussion of the potential risks of a breech vaginal delivery.
- Choice of pain relief.

What do I do in the 2nd stage of labour?

- Perform an abdominal examination to assess the presentation of the presenting part prior to a vaginal examination.
- Confirm full dilatation of the cervix by vaginal examination and establish the breech presentation.
- Call for help — pull the emergency buzzer.
- When help arrives, clearly communicate what is needed and who else you need to be called.
- Inform the woman and partner of what is happening.
- Position the woman in a semi-recumbent position, with a clear space at the end of the bed.
- Consider the environment — do you have enough room for equipment, additional staff arriving and a place for the resusitaire if needed? Ensure that the room is warm enough.

- Remember: 'Hands off the breech'.
- Allow the breech to descend on its own, guiding the woman accordingly.
- Fetal heart assessment — record the fetal heart for five minutes after a contraction. Continuous fetal heart monitoring is recommended (RCOG 2006).
- Episiotomy is only required where it facilitates delivery (RCOG 2006) — selective, rather than routine.
- Let the baby's legs deliver spontaneously. You can aid delivery if needed, by placing two fingers along the length of thigh, fingertips in the popliteal fossae.
- Gently release any loops of cord as necessary.
- Wrap the baby's body in a warm towel.
- Check the position of the baby's arms.
- Keep the baby's back to the mother's front.
- Allow descent of the head to the suboccipital region.
- Promote slow delivery of the head with either the Burns Marshall or the Mauriceau Smellie Veit manoeuvre (Robbins 2011).
- Be prepared to resuscitate the baby.
- Keep the baby warm.
- Encourage early feeding of the baby.
- The baby must be seen and examined by the paediatrician.
- The woman and partner must be debriefed to explain what has occurred.
- Document everything, detailing all of the manoeuvres applied and the times at which events occurred.

References

Barclay L, Kent D (1998) Recent immigration and the misery of motherhood: a discussion of pertinent issues. *Midwifery* **14(1):** 4-9

Barnett BEW, Matthey S, Boyce P (1999) Migration and motherhood: a response to Barclay and Kent *Midwifery* **15(3):** 203-7

Berthoud R (2000) *Family Formation in Multicultural Britain: Three Patterns of Diversity.* ISER Working Papers Paper 2000-34 University of Essex, Colchester. http://www.iser.com ac.uk/pubs/workpaps/pdf/2000-34.pdf (accessed December 2008)

Blaaka G and Eri TS (2008) Doing Midwifery between Different Belief Systems. *Midwifery* **24(3):** 344-352

Bowler I (1993) 'They're not the same as us': midwives' stereotypes of South Asian descent maternity patients. *Sociology of Health and Illness* **15(2):** 157-178

Bryar RM (1995) *Theory for Midwifery Practice.* MacMillan Press Ltd, London

Buckland SS, Homer CSE (2007) Estimating blood loss after birth using simulated clinical examples. Journal of the Australian College of *Midwives* **20(2):** 85-8

Centre for Maternal and Child Enquiries (CMACE) (2007) *Saving Mothers' Lives 2003-2005.* CMACE, London

Cullum A (2009) Weight Management During and After Pregnancy. *Br J Midwifery* **17(6):** 367-8

Davis DL, Walker K (2008) Re-discovering the material body in midwifery through an exploration of theories of embodiment. *Midwifery* **26(4):** 457-62

Directgov (2011) Equality Act 2010. www.directgov.uk (accessed 21/3/11)

Essat Z (2010) *Zenana: The Birth Stories of Migrant Women in Britain.* PhD Thesis (unpublished). De Montfort University, Leicester

Foresight (2007) Tackling Obesities: Future Choices. www.bis.gov.uk/assets/bispartners/ foresight/docs/obesity/17.pdf p34 (accessed 10/12/10)

Hall J (2001) *Midwifery, Mind and Spirit.* Books for Midwives Press, Oxford

Heslehurst N, Ellis L, Simpson H et al (2007) Trends in Maternal Obesity Incidence Rates, Demographic Predictors and Health Inequalities in 36821 women over a 15-year period. *BJOG* **114(2):** 187-194

Holloway I, Wheeler S (2002) *Qualitative Research in Nursing. 2nd edn.* Wiley-Blackwell, London.

Levy V, Moore J (1985) The midwife's management of the third stage of labour. *Nurs Times* **81(39):** 47-50

Lewis G (ed) (2007) The Confidential Enquiry into Maternal and Child Health (CEMACH). *Saving Mothers Lives: reviewing maternal deaths to make motherhood safer 2003-2005. The Seventh Report on Confidential Enquiries into Maternal Death in the United Kingdom.* CEMACH, London

Modder J, Fitzsimons K (2010) *Management of Women with Obesity.* Joint Guideline: CMACE/RCOG

Mousa HA, Alfirevic Z (2007) Treatment for primary postpartum haemorrhage. *Cochrane Database Syst Rev* (1): CD003249.DOI:10.1002?14651858.CD003249.pub2

National Obesity Observatory (NOO) (2010) www.noo.org.uk/NOO_obesity/maternal_obesity/epidemiology (accessed 10/12/10).

NHS Legal Authority (NHLSA) (2010) CNST Maternity Standards 2010/11. www.nhlsa.com (accessed 22 November 2010)

Prasertcharoensuk W, Swanpanich H, Lumbiganon P (2000) Accuracy of the blood loss estimation in the third stage of labor. *Int J Gynecol Obstet.* **71(1):** 69-70

Richens Y, Lavender T (eds) (2010) *Care for Pregnant Women who are Obese.* MA Healthcare, London.

Robbins J (2011) Malpresentation and Malpositions. Ch 6 in Boyle, M (2011) *Emergencies around childbirth.* Radcliffe Publishing, London

Royal College of Obstetricians and Gynaecologists (RCOG) (2009) *Prevention and management of postpartum haemorrhage (Green-top 52).* RCOG, London

Royal College of Obstetricians and Gynaecologists (RCOG) (2006) *Breech presentation and management (Green-top 20b).* www.rcog.org.uk (accessed 21/3/11)

Royal College of Obstetrics and Gynaecologists (RCOG) (2005) *Green Top Guideline 42* www.rcog.org.uk (accessed 31/12/10)

Royston E, Armstrong S (eds) (1989) *Preventing Maternal Deaths.* WHO, Geneva

Soltani H (2009) Obesity in Pregnancy: an evidence-based commentary. *Evidence Based Midwifery* **7(4);** 140 2

World Health Organisation (WHO) (2005) Obesity and Overweight: Factsheet 311. www.who.int/mediacentre/factsheets/fs311/en/ (accessed 10/12/10).

World Health Organisation (WHO) (2002) *Obesity: Preventing and Managing the Global Epidemic.* WHO, Geneva

World Health Organisation (WHO) (1990) *The Prevention and Management of Postpartum Haemorrhage Report of A Technical Working Group.* WHO, Geneva

Chapter 6: Dealing with the unexpected

- **How do I deal with difficult questions?**
- **How do I deal with complaints?**
- **What is involved in incident reporting?**
- **What are my responsibilities in reporting malpractice?**
- **What can I do about bullying within the maternity services?**
- **How do I deal with healthcare associated infections?**

How do I deal with difficult questions?

Jacqui Williams/Kevin Power

Once qualified, it is easy to think that you should 'know everything', regardless of your level of experience (Lathlean 1987; Shand 1987; Power 1996). It is unreasonable to expect anybody to know all of the answers to all of the questions that may be asked.

Most difficult questions will likely fall into one of two categories:

- Questions that you do not know the answer to.
- Questions that you are not sure how to answer.

The first type is relatively easy to deal with. There should be no shame in admitting that you are temporarily unable to answer a question. However, you must promise the woman that you will find out the answer for her, or find another person who can help, and it is important that you keep this promise.

The second type tends to be more challenging as it may need a clear explanation of midwifery and obstetric terms using everyday words. Some questions may also have an ethical component, which needs careful discussion.

Where an answer is technically complex, it can be challenging to ensure that your explanation is understood. Box 6.1 gives an example of such a scenario. You will have to build up a personal 'thesaurus' of everyday words that mean the same as or that explain technical jargon. In many clinical situations, you will need to have a range of explanations to hand, so that you can readily and simply explain situations to both the woman and her partner, avoiding unnecessary worry and anxiety. You can also provide the woman and her partner with written leaflets to read following the discussion, to promote their understanding of the subject.

Where questions have an ethical consideration a direct response is not easy, as there may be a number of answers that can be given to the same question. An example scenario is presented in Box 6.2.

Women will sometimes already know the answers to their questions but they will ask anyway, to seek confirmation. An honest and truthful answer may not come as a shock to the woman. However, this does not mean she will not become upset. You must be prepared to offer appropriate comfort in such situations.

Where you find yourself unable to answer a person's questions, it is not uncommon to be further asked, 'Why, because you don't know or because you

---

Box 6.1 Case Study 1

Following a normal delivery you ask Anisha, who does not have English as her first language, for consent to give vitamin K to her newborn baby. She questions the necessity of giving her baby a 'drug' and asks you if it is safe. She says she has no prior knowledge of vitamin K and she wants her husband to be informed.

Consider the issues here:
• Is this the most appropriate time to have this detailed discussion?
• Is Anisha's English good enough to give informed consent?
• She does not have any prior knowledge of this drug.

Discussions of this nature should be held antenatally with plenty of time for consideration of the issues. If necessary an interpreter should be used and information given in their own language.

On the issue of safety, a balanced approach should be adopted, presenting the arguments for and against its use. Ultimately, the parents will have to decide whether or not they are willing to give consent.

MIDIRS Informed Choice series can be very helpful in this area of practice (www.midirs.org.uk).

don't want to tell me?' A reasonable response here is that you are not the best person to ask and that you will arrange for them to speak with another person who can answer their questions effectively. You must always follow this up, to ensure that both the woman and her partner have all the information they need to make an informed decision.

Box 6.2 Case Study 2

Following raised markers on her maternal serum Down's syndrome screening test, Samantha (aged 27) is due to have an amniocentesis, which will be performed in two days' time.

As her midwife, she asks you about whether or not she will be expected to have a termination of pregnancy if Down's syndrome is detected.

While the answer to this question is 'no', a number of issues must be explored with Samantha and her partner. Discussion will require sensitivity and knowledge about their personal beliefs and values.

In any event, the outcomes are not absolute, so the discussion will take place with a lot of unknown facts about the fetus.

Issues that might be raised:

• How much do Samantha and her partner know about Down's syndrome?
• How severely might the baby affected?
• Do they hold any religious beliefs?
• Are there any siblings?
• What support and help do they have from others in their family?

How do I deal with complaints?

Kevin Power/Jacqui Williams

In the report for 2007–2008, the Parliamentary and Health Service Ombudsman stated that complaints about care are often aggravated by the way in which they are dealt with:

> *Poor complaint handling by NHS bodies and individuals was a recurrent theme across our health investigations in 2007–08'*
> *(Parliamentary and Health Service Ombudsman 2009).*

If not dealt with properly, a complaint that begins as a minor issue can become a major confrontation. Thus, at the very beginning of the process, the way in which a midwife deals with a complaint can have a significant effect on the outcome.

The simplest way to deal with complaints is to prevent them occurring in the first place. Be on the lookout for signs that a woman or relative is becoming irritated — do not wait for the complaint. Ask if there is a problem and if there is, demonstrate to the woman and her partner that you will do your best to deal with it straight away. If this situation is ignored, it is highly likely that a formal complaint will be lodged.

No matter how high your standards of care, or how good your communication skills, it is highly unlikely that the health service will please all of the people all of the time. Patients and their relatives may be anxious or in pain and they are certainly in a strange environment. Additionally, there are high pressures on staff, with heavy workloads and staff shortages. There are always likely to be complaints of one kind or another.

Most NHS Trusts actively seek feedback from patients and service users as part of clinical governance (Robotham 2001). This can enable trusts to forestall complaints through improvements to the service but it can also encourage more people to complain. Each Trust will have protocols and policies in place for dealing with formal complaints and you should be familiar with these. For the purposes of this section, let us focus on those situations where a relative or patient makes a verbal complaint to you.

Think of a time when you have complained about something:

- What was the cause of the complaint?
- Who did you complain to?
- How was the complaint dealt with?
- How did this make you feel?

Most complaints are fairly mundane, but no matter how trivial they may seem to the midwife, all are important to the complainant. The response of the person that is complained to can have a great impact on how far the complainant wants to take the matter, and the level of redress expected. So how does the midwife receiving a verbal complaint respond?

The Wilson Report (DoH 1994) identified several lessons from the private sector:

- **Complainants want an apology, even if the organisation was not at fault** — this does not mean accepting responsibility for the problem. Just saying sorry that the person feels there is a problem can show that you are at least acknowledging their concerns.
- **Complainants want a speedy response** — show that you are willing to take action immediately, even if this is just making time to listen to the complaint. This is difficult when you are busy, but making the complainant wait or passing them on to a more senior member of staff can escalate the situation (Robotham 2001; Parliamentary and Health Service Ombudsman 2009).
- **Complainants want reassurance that the matter is being taken seriously and that the organisation will try to prevent a recurrence** — You should inform complainants what you intend to do about their complaint and how the Trust will respond.
- **Complainants do not want to be told:**
  That rules were being followed, so the organisation was right all along
  - That they made a mistake, so it is their own fault
  - Detailed explanations of why a problem arose, which come across as an excuse for poor services.

It should be your objective to resolve a complaint at the first point of contact — in the first instance, try to handle it yourself. Find out whether or not your employer provides training on complaints handling and ask to be sent for some if it is offered. You should prepare yourself as best you can to deal with complaints as they arise. If, after listening carefully, it becomes clear that you cannot resolve the issue, or if the complaint is a serious one, you should inform the complainant about how they can take the matter further.

If this is the first time you have had to deal with a complaint, you should seek support from the senior midwife on duty or your Supervisor of Midwives, your senior nurse or duty manager. You will not be expected to deal with a complaint by yourself, and more senior staff will expect to be involved. Also, no matter how competently you deal with a complaint, some people will not be satisfied until they have spoken to someone 'in authority'. If your situation seems to be heading this way, do not see it as a failure — swallow your pride and call in a suitable member of staff.

Finally, do not forget to record the complaint and the action you have taken in the midwifery notes. Even if you feel that the complaint was dealt with immediately and the matter has been resolved, the complainant may want to take things further at a later date. Clear records of the complaint, the time/date and the outcome will be vital if a formal investigation takes place. You must also complete an incident form.

What is involved in incident reporting!

Kevin Power/Jacqui Williams

In 2008–2009, the NHS paid out £226 million for obstetrics and gynaecology maternity negligence claims (NHSLA 2009). Negligence claims against the NHS remain at high levels — in 2009–2010, the NHS Litigation Authority (NHSLA) received 6088 claims for clinical negligence (resulting in £787 million being paid out) and 4074 for non-clinical negligence. Obstetrics and gynaecology maternity claims remain the highest (NHSLA 2010).

Your immediate response to an incident is important. Clearly, the priority is to ensure that anyone who is hurt receives prompt attention for their injuries. Where an incident occurs that may lead to a claim being made against a midwife, seek prompt advice from both your Supervisors of Midwives and your professional union e.g. the Royal College of Midwives.

Green (2001) notes that there is some confusion over how to respond when an incident occurs and advises that practitioners should not rush to apologise for an incident but should instead record the facts, ensure that the line manager is promptly made aware of the incident, and cooperate with the complaints procedure. Green (2001) argues that an appropriate point at which to apologise is on completion of the investigation, when there is no longer the risk of compromising any indemnity insurance you may have. However, the NHSLA (2009) states that expressing sorrow or regret when something has happened does not constitute an admission of liability, therefore sympathising with the woman is not necessarily inappropriate.

All incidents that lead to harm, whether major or minor, must be reported (DoH 2001). You must also report any 'near misses' — incidents that nearly lead to harm. Each employer will have local systems in place for reporting incidents and near misses, and you should become familiar with those in your area.

The minimum requirements for recording of incidents are listed below.

What do I write?

- Write your full name, your qualifications and when gained, your job title, your employer's address and how long you have been working there at the time of the incident.
- Write how you were involved in the incident — for example, you may have been the midwife on duty, caring for the woman at the time.
- Write why you are writing the statement — who has asked you to write the statement and why? Give a brief description.
- When writing the record it is important to note clear and unambiguous facts — give a factual narrative of the your role in the woman's care.
- State what you saw or what others say they saw, not what you or they think happened. For example, if a woman is found on the floor in the bathroom, do not write 'she seemed to have fallen while taking a shower' — instead, write 'she was found lying on the floor in the bathroom'. You can record what someone says, e.g. 'Kate Jackson stated that she felt faint getting in the shower and went down onto the floor.'
- Where you do record what someone says, it is important to make clear that you are using another person's words by enclosing their statement in quotation marks.
- Write events in the order in which they occurred — you will need to refer to the patient notes. If you are recording things from memory, you must state this. You may refer to any guidelines that were in place at the time.
- Everything you write should be factual, not based on opinion. Explain any terminology that might not be familiar to a layperson.
- Include anything that was happening at the time in the practice setting where the incident occurred. For example, were there sufficient midwives on duty? Was it very busy? Was it a bank holiday? Were you new to the area?
- State who else was involved in the woman's care, by name if you can.
- State how you respond to any allegations that are made against you.
- Comment on when your involvement with the woman ceased, e.g. when you handed over to another midwife.
- Number all the pages and paragraphs. Check that the statement is free from grammatical errors and spelling mistakes.
- Each page of the statement should be signed and name printed. Keep a copy of the statement in a safe place, in case you need to refer to it.
- Write down the events in chronological order, to help clarify precisely what happened. All witnesses should make a statement — if the witness is another woman, a relative or a junior member of staff, they may need advice on how to write what happened, to ensure that they also report facts rather than opinion.

(Adapted from 'Guidance on Statement Writing' RCM 2008)

If the woman was injured or there is a suspicion of injury as a result of the incident, a doctor should examine her and record all the findings.

It is often useful to write some personal notes after an event, in case you need to write a statement later. Alongside the notes, this will help you to write an accurate account.

What are my responsibilities in reporting malpractice?
Kevin Power/Jacqui Williams

'Negligence: failure to act with the prudence that a reasonable person would exercise under the same circumstances; lack of due care, omission of duty, habitual neglect'

(Webster's Dictionary 2010)

Hall et al (2010) suggest that a midwife is negligent when she acts in a careless way and causes injury to a mother or baby. It can be argued that this can be extended to cover all practice that has the potential to cause injury. Hall and colleagues further suggest that true test is what most midwives would do in the same situation.

The Nursing and Midwifery Council (NMC) reminds us that midwives have a professional obligation to report concerns in the workplace (NMC 2010). The NMC has produced guidance, which supports midwives in the effective management of risk and that empowers them to speak out.

There are two types of situation that may lead you to report malpractice:

- Malpractice specifically relating to practitioners whose names appear on a professional register, such as midwives and doctors — usually termed 'professional misconduct'.
- Malpractice by anyone else within the area of care, or concerns about poor standards.

Professional misconduct

Table 6.3 lists the most common types of professional misconduct reported to the NMC.

Table 6.3. The most common types of professional misconduct allegations reported to the NMC

	2007–2008	2008–2009
Dishonesty*	17.32%	14.83%
Patient abuse (physical, sexual, verbal inappropriate relationship)	14.30%	8.37%
Failure to maintain adequate records	10.37%	8.52%
Incorrect administration of drugs	9.87%	11.75%
Neglect of basic care	9 16%	10.57%
Unsafe clinical practice	7.75%	7.78%
Failure to collaborate with colleagues	6.95%	6.9%
Colleague abuse (physical, sexual, verbal, inappropriate relationship)	2.72%	1.9%
Failure to report incidents	2.62%	0.44%
Failure to act in an emergency	1.91%	2.06%
Pornography — adult	1.01%	0.59%

*Dishonesty includes theft, fraud, false claim to registration, claiming sick pay fraudulently, falsification of records, dishonesty about previous employment and misappropriation of drugs. (NMC 2009)

You need to be sure of your facts and give a clear factual account of your concerns — this means stating what has actually occurred rather than what you suspect may have occurred. If you can get other witnesses to support you, all the better. If there are no other witnesses, you should still make sure to record all of the facts, including the date and time and precisely what you observed. Remember — write down what you saw, not what you think happened.

Many staff are afraid to report malpractice and poor standards because of the potential for recriminations and possibly even job loss (O'Dowd 2002). Certainly, the students that the author teaches often say they would feel uncomfortable complaining about poor standards of care, in case it influences the assessment by the mentor at the end of the placement. This culture of fear of reprisal seems to persist for qualified staff (Nazarko 1998; Health Which 1999; Wallis 2001; Ferns and Chojnacka 2005), despite the enactment of the Public Interest Disclosure Act 1998, which protects the whistleblower if victimised or dismissed as a result of disclosing malpractice.

Your fitness to practice may be questioned if you do comply with the NMC Code (2008), which is clear of a midwife's responsibility to report concerns.

Raising a concern, or making a complaint?

The NMC (2010) clarifies the difference between a concern and a complaint:

- A **concern** is when you are worried about an issue that affects others and you want you to protect them. Your employer will have a whistleblowing policy to protect those who raise concerns.
- You may wish to make a **complaint** about how you are being treated at work. Here you use your employer's complaints and grievance procedure.

The NMC Code (2008) stipulates that:

- You must act without delay if you believe that you, a colleague or anyone else may be putting someone at risk.
- You must inform someone in authority if you experience problems that prevent you working within the code or other nationally agreed standards*.
- You must report your concerns in writing if problems in the environment or care are putting people at risk**

*For example, NICE Guidelines.
**Your Supervisor of Midwives, your mentor, or university tutor.

Steps to follow

- Check your employer's whistleblowing policy.
- Review the NMC guidance ('Raising and escalating concerns: guidance for nurses and midwives' 2010).
- Receive appropriate support and advice from your professional body, e.g. the Royal College of Midwives.
- Raise your concerns internally.

- Keep a clear record of any written or verbal communication that you send or receive from your employer, respecting confidentiality.
- Agree a timeframe for action with your employer.
- Escalate your concerns internally, outside your management line if the timeframe has been breached or you are not happy with the response, e.g. department manager, Head of Midwifery.
- Following advice from your professional body, you may 'go public'

(Adapted from 'Raising and escalating concerns: Guidance for nurses and midwives', NMC 2010)

Will I be protected if I raise a concern?

The Public Interest Disclosure Act (1988) (PIDA) was introduced to protect those who honestly raise concerns about issues in practice, and this protects you.
For more information, visit:
http://pcaw.co.uk/law/uklegislation.htm

Whistle-blowing advice

- Stay calm.
- Remember that you are a witness, and not a complainant.
- Think about the risks and outcomes before you act.
- Let the facts speak for themselves — don't make ill-considered allegations.
- Remember that you may be mistaken, or that there may be an innocent or good explanation.
- Do not become a private detective.
- Recognise that you may not be thanked.

(Public Concern at Work 2009)

What does the Health Service Ombudsman do?

The Health Service Ombudsman (HSO) provides a service for members of the public to complain about hospitals and a range of health professionals. Should a complaint not be successfully resolved within a Trust or practice, they will assess whether or not they can handle the complaint. Where they have the legal power to do so, they undertake independent investigations into complaints that the NHS has not acted properly on.

For more information, visit:

http://www.ombudsman.org.uk/

What can I do about bullying within the maternity services?

Kevin Power/Jacqui Williams

Bullying is increasingly being recognised as a problem. During a confidential investigation in her own maternity unit, O'Brien (2011) found that as a result of bullying, 80% of her staff reported being physically sick on at least one occasion before coming to work. Many midwives spoke of being treated badly by their peers, which Leap (1997) describes as 'horizontal bullying.' The same investigation found that three senior midwives were perpetrators of bullying.

The Royal College of Midwives (RCM) supports the need for a 'Dignity at Work Bill', which would give more protection to employees who are being bullied in the workplace — this is particularly needed as currently many midwives may fear possible reprisals for reporting bullying.

As a midwife, you have a professional duty to take action if you are aware that someone is being bullied. Although the NMC Code of Professional Conduct (NMC 2008) does not make explicit mention of bullying, it does state that there is a duty to report circumstances in the care environment that could jeopardise standards of practice. It would be hard to imagine anyone delivering a high standard of care if they were subject to bullying. Your employer will probably also place a duty on you, through local policies, to take action if you are aware of bullying. So how do you recognise when you or another member of staff is being bullied? It is not always obvious when you are being bullied.

Howells-Johnson (2000) defines bullying as 'persistent unwelcome behaviour', such as:

- Unwarranted or invalid criticism.
- Nit-picking.
- Fault finding.
- Exclusion.
- Isolation of another.
- Singling someone out.
- Treating someone differently.
- Shouting at someone.
- Humiliating someone.
- Excessive monitoring of someone's work performance.

Other examples include making unreasonable work demands of a person and inciting others to hold a negative opinion of someone.

What should you do?

The first thing to do is to recognise bullying behaviour for what it is. There can be no excuse for it, especially in the workplace. Any criticism of your or anyone else's performance should be constructive and based on facts, not destructive and based on conjecture. As with much of what is discussed in this chapter, record what is happening. According to Grove (2000) it is not the incident itself that necessarily counts, but the frequency and the regularity with which it happens. White (2002a) suggests talking to colleagues about the bullying, as you may not be the only one. Talking to others may reveal several team members who do not like the situation, and who are prepared to support you in taking action against the bully.

Your trust or employer should have anti-bullying policies in place. Find out what they are and use them to take action. Dimond (2002) points out that your employer has a legal duty under health and safety law to protect employees from bullying. Additionally, under Article 3 of the Human Rights Act 1998, you have the right to freedom from inhuman and degrading treatment. It is inhuman and degrading to bully someone and the employer has a clear duty to prevent this abuse of human rights. You also have legal protection under the Public Interest Disclosure Act 1998 if you blow the whistle and report an employer for bullying (see section on reporting malpractice).

You should be aware of the negative effects that bullying can have on health and if you feel that your health is affected, you should seek medical advice. If you have time off sick as a result of bullying, record it in the accident book at work. If necessary, you can take out a grievance against the bully through your employer's grievance procedures. Human resources or personnel departments should be able to give advice and support in this. Your union representative should also be able to offer advice and guidance on handling the situation.

Several case studies of bullying reported in the press have revealed that victims can feel embarrassed about being victims and suffer in silence until they are driven out of their jobs. The key is to not suffer alone but to share your feelings with others and report bullying behaviour. Grove (2000) goes so far as to suggest that if a bully is aggressive in public, you should get a solicitor's letter sent to them. You must not let the bully force a change in your behaviour or cause you to move jobs — not only will your self-esteem take a serious blow, but the bully is likely to move on to another target. You should not have to pay the price for another person's unacceptable behaviour.

How do I deal with healthcare associated infections?
Kevin Power/Jacqui Williams

Healthcare associated infections (HAIs) are infections that are acquired as a result of healthcare interventions. They lead to longer hospital stays and can be life-threatening. Antibiotic-resistant bacteria are a constant worry in the health service and the media regularly reports the outbreak of 'superbugs'. How should we be dealing with this problem?

Accounting for 20% of all HAIs, urinary tract infections (UTIs) are the second largest group of HAIs in the UK (HPA 2009). As well as being potentially painful and even life-threatening, these infections can lead to preterm delivery and as a result, potentially low birth weight babies (NICE 2008). As the rate of lower segment caesarean section increases and more women need to be catheterised in a maternity setting, this is of particular concern to midwives.

The key message here for the midwife is to ensure that the urine is routinely tested at antenatal visits and that prompt action is taken if proteinuria is detected. Bladder care must be promoted in labour and if catheterisation becomes necessary, a strict aseptic technique must be adopted and the catheter must be vigilantly monitored when *in situ* to identify early any signs of infection.

Meticillin-resistant *Staphylococcus aureus* (MRSA) and *Clostridium difficile* (*C. diff*) are the two most significant causative agents but this should not obscure the fact that there are many potential sources of infection both in healthcare institutions and in the home.

Box 6.4 Management of suspected *C. diff.* infection

The Department of Health (2009) recommends the following:

• All staff should apply the following mnemonic protocol (SIGHT) when managing suspected, potentially infectious diarrhoea:

S: Suspect that a case may be infective where there is no clear alternative cause for diarrhoea.

I: Isolate the woman and consult with the Infection Control Team (ICT) while determining the cause of the diarrhoea.

G: Gloves and aprons must be used for all contacts with the woman and her environment.

H: Hand-washing with soap and water should be carried out before and after each contact with the woman and her environment.

T: Test the stool for toxin, by sending a specimen immediately.

• Always wash your hands after you have had any physical contact with a woman. Do not rely solely on alcohol gel — this does not kill *C. difficile* spores.
• If you suspect infection, a simple diagnostic test can be done to see if *C. difficile* toxins are present in a sample of diarrhoeal faeces, giving a result within a few hours. During outbreaks, or when monitoring the different strains circulating in the population, *C. difficile* can be cultured from faeces and isolates can then be sent to the Anaerobe Reference Laboratory (National Public Health Service, Cardiff) or to HPA regional laboratories for typing and testing for antibiotic susceptibility.
• Women with infections should be isolated and the health professionals caring for them should wear gloves and aprons, especially when dealing with bedpans, etc.
• Environments should be kept clean at all times. Where there are cases of *C. difficile* infection, a disinfectant containing chlorine or other sporicidal agent should be used to reduce environmental contamination.

Box 6.5 Management of suspected *MRSA* infection

The following is adapted from the Department of Health (DoH) (2007) advice sheet. For more detailed information, see the DoH website: www.dh.gov.uk

To reduce the likelihood of spreading infection you should:

• Always wash your hands or use an antibacterial hand rub after you have had any physical contact with a woman — whether or not the woman has a wound. Remember that midwives can be carriers of the bacteria even if they are not infected themselves.
• Encourage women to wash their hands after using the toilet, prior to handling the baby and before and after eating.
• If you suspect infection, take a swab or another sample from the suspected infection site and send it for laboratory analysis.
• If a woman is infected, always use gloves when caring for her and isolate her from other mothers, to prevent the bacteria spreading.

Final points

In addition to familiarising yourself with the management of suspected MRSA and *C. diff.* infections (see boxes 6.4 and 6.5), you should ensure that you are up to date with the current advice regarding swine flu and pregnancy, as this has been changing slightly year on year.

Remember that if a woman is labelled 'infectious' and confined to a side room, she is likely to feel isolated and possibly stigmatised. You can help the woman by encouraging visitors to stagger the times of their visits. Make sure that the woman understands her condition and that she is not isolated unless absolutely necessary. All trusts have an infection control nurse or team and they will be an invaluable source of information and support to the ward staff and the woman. Lastly, do not forget that she will need the same support and advice as any new mother.

References

Department of Health (DOH) (2011) Seasonal Flu Jab. www.dh.gov.uk (accessed 25/2/11)

Department of Health (DOH) (2009) Clostridium difficile: how to deal with the problem. www.dh.gov.uk (accessed 25/2/11)

Department of Health (DOH) (2007) A simple guide to MRSA. www.dh.gov.uk (accessed 25/2/11)

Department of Health (DOH) (2004) *Being Heard: the report of a review committee on NHS complaints procedures (Wilson Report)*. HMSO, London

Department of Health (DOH) (2001) *Building a safer NHS for patients: implementing an organisation with a memory*. HMSO, London

Dimond B (2002) Workplace stress and bullying: liabilities of the employer. *Br J Nurs.* **11(10):** 699-701

Ferns T, Chojnocko I (2005) Reporting incidents of violence and aggression towards NHS staff. *Nurs Stand.* **19(38):** 51-6

Georgiou G (2007) Anti-bullying tactics make a difference. *RCM Midwives* **10(6):** 268

Green C (2001) Benefiting from the end of blame culture. *Prof Nurse* **16(7 suppl.):** S3-4

Grove J (2000) Survival and resistance. *Nurs Times* **96(18):** 26-8

Hall H, McKenna L, Griffiths D (2010) Understanding negligence as a crime in midwifery. *Br J Midwifery* **18(7):** 350-8

Health Protection Agency (2009) *Trends in rates of healthcare associated infection in England 2004-2008*, NAO, London

Health Which? (1999) Blowing the whistle. *Health Which? April:* 16-7

Howells-Johnson J (2000) Verbal abuse. *Br J Perioper Nurs,* **10(10):** 508-511

Human Rights Act (1998) Equality and Human Rights Commission. www.equalityhumanrights.com (accessed 13/3/11)

Lathlean J (1987) Are you prepared to be a staff nurse? *Nurs Times* **83(36):** 25 7

Leap N (1997) Making sense of 'horizontal violence' in midwifery. *Br J Midwifery* **5(11):** 689

MIDIRS (2011) Informed Choice leaflets. www.midirs.org.uk

National Institute for Health and Clinical Excellence (2008) *Antenatal Care routine care for the healthy pregnant woman*. www.nice.org.uk (accessed 25/2/11) RCOG, London

Nazarko L (1998) Breaking the silence. *Elder Care.* **10(3):** 44

National Health Service Litigation Authority (NHSLA) (2010) Report and Accounts 2010. www.nhsla.com (accessed 13/3/11)

National Health Service Litigation Authority (NHSLA) (2009) Report and Accounts 2009. www.nhsla.com (accessed 13/3/11)

National Health Service Litigation Authority (NHSLA) (2009) Dear Colleague Letter May 1. www.nhsla.com (accessed 13/3/11)

Nursing and Midwifery Council (NMC) (2010) *Raising and escalating concerns Guidance for nurses and midwives.* NMC, London

Nursing and Midwifery Council (NMC) (2008) *The code: Standards of conduct and performance and ethics for nurses and midwives.* NMC, London

Nursing and Midwifery Council (NMC) (2004) *Midwives rules and standards.* NMC, London

O'Brien M (2011) Bullying in midwifery. www.rcm.org.uk (accessed 10/3/2011)

Parliamentary and Health Service Ombudsman (2009) 2007 08 Annual report. www.cfps.org.uk (accessed 19/10/10)

Pearce L (2001) Bully at work. *Nurs Standard* **15(27):** 14-15

Power K (1996) *First time practice as children's nurse: A phenomenological inquiry.* Unpublished dissertation, De Montfort University, Leicester

Public Concern at Work (2009) How do I blow the whistle? www.pcaw.co.uk/faq

Public Interest Disclosure Act (1998) www.legislation.gov.uk (accessed 13/3/11)

Robotham, M. (2001) How to handle complaints. *Nurs Times* **97(30):** 25-8

Royal College of Midwives (2007) Guidance to statement writing London. www.rcm.org.uk (accessed 10/311)

Shand M (1997) Unreasonable expectations. *Nurs Times* **83(36):** 28-30

Wallis L (2001) Protecting the whistle blower. *Nurs Standard* **13(47):** 16-7

Webster's 1913 Dictionary (2010) www.webster-dictionary.org/definition/negligence (accessed 25/2/11)

White, C. (2002) The enemy within. *Nurs Times* **98(44):** 12-3

Index